The CIVAS Handbook

Richard Needle

Richard Needle graduated with a BPharm from Bath University in 1978. After a preregistration year at Peterborough District Hospital, he returned to Bath to undertake a PhD in Synthetic and Analytical Organic Chemistry. In 1982 he joined the Pharmacy Department at Queens Medical Centre as a basic grade pharmacist before moving on to Colchester at the beginning of 1984. His first post at Colchester was Staff Pharmacist, Radiopharmacy, charged also with the setting up of the cytotoxic service. He has had several posts in Colchester over the succeeding years but his remit has always included aseptic services. In February 1997 he was appointed Chief Pharmacist for Essex Rivers Healthcare NHS Trust, based at Colchester General Hospital.

Richard Needle was a member of the Cytotoxic Services Working Party throughout its existence and is a contributor to the *Cytotoxics Handbook*. As CIVAS developed in the late 1980s, he saw that a similar group would be of value in this area. He was instrumental in the launch of the National CIVAS Group in 1992 and has been Chairman of the Group since its inception. He has represented the Group on a number of special committees since that time. Richard also maintains a clinical interest in oncology and palliative care.

Tim Sizer

Tim Sizer began his career as an industrial chemist, but went on to obtain a BPharm(Hons) degree from Chelsea College, University of London in 1977. He followed this with a preregistration year in Westminster Hospital and three years at the Royal Free Hospital, confirming his interest in hospital pharmacy and pharmaceutical preparation. In 1981, he moved to Cheltenham to manage a sub-regional sterile production unit specialising in the preparation of intravenous solutions in PVC containers. In the course of his time at Cheltenham, he re-developed the sterile and aseptic services to include cytotoxic reconstitution, special eye-drop preparation and TPN compounding, the latter being supplied to hospitals throughout the UK.

Tim Sizer is currently the Technical Services Manager for the Charing Cross and Hammersmith Hospitals, and is responsible for the activities of two large aseptic suites and a busy non-sterile production facility. He maintains an active interest in clinical nutritional support, intensive care medicine, oncology, and all aspects of pharmaceutical formulation.

He is the chairman of the British Pharmaceutical Nutrition Group (formerly the National TPN Group) and has been a leading member of the National CIVAS Group since its inception. He is a council member of the British Association for Parenteral & Enteral Nutrition and has participated in numerous national working parties including the Kings Fund 'A positive approach to nutrition as treatment' (1992). He was editor and contributor to 'Standards and guidelines for nutritional support of patients in hospitals' (BAPEN 1996). He has lectured widely and is a part-time lecturer for the University of Leeds.

The CIVAS Handbook

The centralised intravenous additive services reference

Edited by

Richard Needle
BPharm, PhD, MRPharmS
Chief Pharmacist
Colchester General Hospital
Colchester, UK.

and

Tim Sizer
BPharm, MRPharmS
Principal Pharmacist Technical Services
Hammersmith Hospital
London, UK.

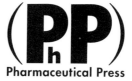

Pharmaceutical Press

Published by the Pharmaceutical Press
1 Lambeth High Street, London SE1 7JN

First published 1998

© 1998 Pharmaceutical Press

Printed in Great Britain at The University Press, Cambridge

ISBN 0 85369 396 X

A catalogue record for this book is available from the British Library

Contents

CIVAS Contributors

Brian Baker
Pharmacy Department, Royal Free Hospital, London

Mike Booth
Pharmacy Department, Stepping Hill Hospital, Stockport

Steve Brown
Pharmacy Department, Bristol Royal Infirmary, Bristol

Martin Callam
Pharmacy Department, Norfolk and Norwich Hospital, Norwich

Amanda Carthew
Pharmacy Department, Northwick Park & St Mark's NHS Trust, Harrow, Middlesex

Christine Clarke
Pharmacy Department, Leicester Royal Infirmary, Leicester

Krissy Cock
Pharmacy Department, West Middlesex University Hospital, Isleworth, Middlesex

Denise Fenton
Pharmacy Department, The Royal Oldham Hospital, Oldham

Charlotte Gibb
Pharmacy Department, Leeds General Infirmary, Leeds

Frank Haines-Nutt
Pharmacy Department, Torbay Hospital, Torquay, Devon

Con Hanson
Pharmacy Department, Ipswich Hospital, Ipswich

Sandra Harding
Pharmacy Department, Oxford Radcliffe Hospital, Oxford

John Hubbard
Pharmacy Department, Gloucestershire Royal Hospital, Gloucester

Adele Jones
Pharmacy Department, Gloucestershire Royal Hospital, Gloucester

Suzanne Kendall-Smith
Pharmacy Department, St James University Hospital, Leeds

Jeff Koundakjian
Clatterbridge Hospital, Bebington, Wirral

Martin Lee
Pharmacy Department, Derbyshire Royal Infirmary, Derby

Ian Marsha
Pharmacy Department, Royal South Hampshire Hospital, Southampton

Claire McIntyre
Pharmacy Department, Peterborough District Hospital, Peterborough

Daniel Murphy
Pharmacy Department, Royal London Hospital, London

Richard Needle
Pharmacy Department, Colchester General Hospital, Colchester

Duncan Petty
Pharmacy Department, Leeds General Infirmary, Leeds

Melanie Priston
Pharmacy Research Laboratory, Derriford Hospital, Plymouth

Chris Pritchard
Pharmacy Department, Thanet District General Hospital, Margate

Tim Sizer
Pharmacy Department, Hammersmith Hospital, London

James Thom
Pharmacy Department, Southampton General Hospital, Southampton

Christine Trehane
Pharmacy Department, Royal Free Hospital, London

Paul Weller
Pharmaceutical Press, Royal Pharmaceutical Society of Great Britain, London

Preface

The foundations for the development of centralised intravenous additive services (CIVAS) were laid in the mid 1970s when the working party, chaired by Professor Alisdair Breckenridge, reported in 1976.

The working party met at a time of increasing usage of the intravenous route for drug administration and developing awareness that problems were occurring due to contamination of injections, and incompatible mixtures being prepared. The *Breckenridge Report* recommended that the preparation of intravenous injections was properly a pharmaceutical activity and the responsibility of hospital pharmacy. It is a matter of history that the subsequent development of CIVAS was slow, with very few services being developed for drugs other than cytotoxics and parenteral nutrition for more than ten years.

Widespread development of CIVAS began towards the end of the 1980s and it was in response to this more rapid development that a group of interested hospital pharmacists met in 1991 and formed the National CIVAS Group. The Group took as its remit the formulation and development of good practice guidance, and to disseminate this information to pharmacists interested in setting up a CIVAS, and those who operated them.

In 1993, the National CIVAS Group produced the *CIVAS Manual* which was published by the Group and distributed amongst hospital pharmacists, primarily throughout the UK. The document was well received and many enquiries have been received over the past four years regarding an updated version of that manual. This *CIVAS Handbook* is the successor to the original manual and is updated and expanded in response to the many comments received.

The *CIVAS Handbook*, as before, provides guidance to those who are considering the setting up of a CIVAS. It raises the many and varied issues that need to be considered at the planning stage, follows through with the setting up of operational procedures, the training, and finally, the auditing of the functioning service. The intention of the guidance included in this handbook is to provide a template; a guide on how to approach the setting up and operation of a CIVAS. It is not intended to be comprehensive or prescriptive, but as a body of information that can be adapted to suit local needs and requirements and set appropriate local standards.

The most significant addition from the original manual is the inclusion of drug monographs. Approximately 40 of the most commonly used intravenous drugs have had monographs prepared which draw together much of the salient literature regarding the stability of the drugs. This is designed to guide local decision making regarding the handling of these drug entities within a CIVAS. There is a more detailed introduction to the monograph section (chapter 8) but it is important to bear in mind that there is no substitute for critically appraising the original study work before making decisions on storage conditions and shelf-lives for drugs prepared in a local CIVAS.

The large amount of feedback that was received after the distribution of the *CIVAS Manual* was extremely useful and helped to guide the preparation of this handbook. Once again, the editors would welcome all feedback, both positive and negative, in order to gauge whether future editions of the *CIVAS Handbook* would be justified and how the content should be achieved.

Finally, the editors would like to thank all those whose hard work in preparing the contributed monographs and chapters has made publication of this book possible.

Richard Needle and **Tim Sizer**
Colchester and London, February 1998

1 Setting up a CIVAS

Jeff Koundakjian

1.1 Introduction

In 1974, a series of incidents concerning the use of intravenous infusions led to the setting up of a working party under the chairmanship of Professor Alistair Breckenridge. The *Breckenridge Report*[1] examined all aspects of the addition of drugs to intravenous fluids. It noted the hazards which could arise from microbial contamination due to poor aseptic conditions or technique, the problems of drug incompatibilities, and it recognised that many of the medical and nursing staff involved in this practice had received insufficient training. The report concluded that 'the addition of drugs to intravenous infusion fluid is an aseptic pharmaceutical procedure, which should ideally be carried out in appropriate environmental conditions under the direct control of a pharmacist.'

The recommendations of the report became more relevant as a consequence of the strict liability provisions of the *Consumer Protection Act* which became effective in March 1988.[2] Part 1 of this act states that the authority (or trust) may incur liability for a defective product unless the producer or manufacturer can be identified, and also states that if a product is manipulated in some way e.g. reconstituted, diluted, or added to an infusion, subsequent liability for the safety of the product may be borne by the trust.

A document was released in December 1994, *Aseptic Dispensing for NHS Patients,*[3] which provides the basic framework for the operation of an additive service and draws attention to other current relevant guidance documents. Adherence to, and understanding of, the standards these guidelines demand are necessary for the management of risk.

Before planning a centralised intravenous additive service (CIVAS) there are a number of areas to be studied in order to justify to doctors, nurses, managers, and pharmacy staff, the introduction of such a service. Before proceeding, the following questions should be asked.

What is the current situation?
• What is the workload? Demand will increase.

• What methods are used for prescribing, preparation and administration?
• What response time is required.

What are the problems of the current situation?
• Identify problems and their significance.
• What are the costs (or savings) versus benefits?
In answering these questions, and others, that develop from the assessment process, a good case can be prepared for the establishment and operation of a CIVAS. Some of the benefits that have been considered are as follows.

1.2 Potential Benefits of a CIVAS
The benefits of a CIVAS can be summarised as:
• Drug administration by appropriate method and rate.
• Drug administration at correct time.
• Reduction in medication error.
• Improved formulary compliance.
• Improved pharmacy control.
• Financial reports available.
• Greater pharmacy involvement in intravenous therapy.
• Better health and safety control.
• Comprehensive documentation.
• High assurance of stability and sterility.
• Standardisation of drug concentration and methods of administration.

1.3 Potential Cost Benefits of a CIVAS
• Reduced drug wastage.
• Saving of nurse/doctor preparation time.
• Improved formulary compliance.
• Increased control over ward drug stocks.

1.4 Potential Problems of a CIVAS
• Increased expenditure (e.g. if using commercial services, increased staff and resource costs).
• Communication of requirements.
• Distribution and storage.
• Retrieval and re-use of unused doses.
• Increased staff to satellite units.

- Limited ability to prepare first and 'stat' doses.
- Difficult to service wards and departments requiring unusual drugs and doses rapidly (e.g. A&E, ITUs, theatres).
- Out-of-hours service.
- Capital expenditure in pharmacy.
- Individualised doses (e.g. paediatrics).

In order to estimate the resources likely to be needed to operate a CIVAS, careful consideration of the correct situation is needed. This establishes a baseline against which the success of the CIVAS can be measured and provides an indication of the future workload.

1.5 What is the Current Situation?

Range of service and projected workload

It will be necessary to establish:

- The type of preparations used.
- The number of individual doses administered annually.
- The stability of the preparations administered.
- Who prescribes the parenteral therapy?
- Who prepares the preparation and who administers the drug; is it the same person?
- How long does it take to prepare the preparation in a safe and proper way?
- Can adequate time be allowed for documentation?
- Can wastage be quantified?
- Workload patterns for each ward/department/directorate.
- Ratio of bolus injection to infusion (intermittent or continuous) as method of administration.

Training

- Are doctors and nurses adequately trained to prepare parenteral drugs?

Health and safety

- Are existing arrangements satisfactory and appropriate for patient safety and operator protection?

Cost

- What is the current expenditure in terms of drugs, equipment, facilities and staff?
- Are there sufficient amounts of nursing and medical time which could be better utilised providing direct patient care?

- Can the value of some of the time saved be tied to the pharmacy budget?
- Is drug wastage a significant financial issue (e.g. paediatrics)?
- Will the provision of a centralised service reduce or increase revenue expenditure?

Quality issues

- Check suitability of preparation areas.
- Are there checks on patient, prescription, drug selection, compatibility?
- Administration time versus prescribed time.
- Is the duration of the injection appropriate?
- Are there interruptions?
- Are medication errors documented?
- Are administration methods appropriate?
- Are vial/ampoule contents stored and re-used?
- Is there recording of batch numbers?

1.6 Pilot Schemes

A CIVAS is a major development and will require either additional resources or development of existing resources. Before proceeding further, an awareness of local and district strategic plans is needed, together with an examination of the present level of commitments and resources to ensure that a proper balance of resource commitment is achieved.

A pilot scheme is an effective mechanism of collecting data, canvassing opinion and testing logistics and procedures. A multidisciplinary working party should be established to set clear objectives and a fixed endpoint. A decision, which is then made on whether or not to proceed, is based on local experience.

All interested parties should be consulted for information and opinions on the type of service required and for their support. Any locally identified problems and incidents should be documented in a statement of need. After acceptance of the need it will be useful to set up a working party. Local circumstances will determine its constitution. However, membership of the working party should include representatives from management, pharmacy, nursing staff and clinicians (*see* below).

- Clinicians: representatives of the departments who would be major users of the service.
- Health and safety representative.
- Management: senior operational or directorate business manager.
- Risk manager or member of the risk manage-

ment team.
- Nursing staff: nurse managers and users of the service.
- Pharmacy: pharmacists and technicians.

The objectives of the working party should be:
- To establish and coordinate a pilot study in accordance with previously agreed aims and objectives.
- To assess the capital and revenue implications of a service and allocate resources as appropriate.
- To decide what type of service is required.
- To decide what level of service is required.
- To monitor the performance of the service.
- To formulate policy and to provide advice on relevant issues.

1.7 What Type of Service is Required?

When deciding on the type of service to be provided, certain areas should be considered.

Workload

The volume of work in terms of individual patient doses per annum, annual expenditure on the type of drugs to be used, and the presentation of drugs (e.g. syringes or bags) are key considerations.

Range and presentation of doses

Key areas to consider are:
- The range of doses used.
- The stability of the solutions of the drugs used.
- Methods of administration (bolus injection, intermittent or continuous infusion).
- Is there formulary control of drugs?
- Is there standardisation of doses?
- Are 'stat' doses to be included?
- Are paediatric departments, ITU, A&E, and theatres to be catered for?

Level of service

Determine the level of service pharmacy can provide. Can a total service be provided during normal working hours or does a 24 hour service need to be established? How will 'out-of-hours' requirements be met; will 'on-call' arrangements be required?

If some doses are prepared on the ward, the skill level of staff will need to be addressed since there will be a loss of skills due to the reduction or disappearance of medical and nursing preparation. The preparative skills of the 'on-call' pharmacists also need to be addressed.

Quality assurance and sterility assurance

Quality assurance procedures should be agreed, documented and adhered to. In order to achieve high levels of product assurance, procedures should include rigorous standards for equipment, maintenance, operator training, and environmental monitoring, and action plans for deviations from defined limits.

Licence implications for service

With the removal of crown immunity, careful consideration should be given to whether a licence is required and if not, the staffing requirements needed to fulfil the exemption under section 10 of the *Medicines Act*[4] (*see* section 1.8).

Facilities

Utilise existing facilities if available. If not available convert facilities and purchase appropriate equipment. Consider the merits of isolators versus clean rooms. Seek current guidance on facilities specifications.

Health and safety

Local and national guidelines should be adhered to.

Risk management

A culture of proactive risk management must be in place with clear guidelines and procedures, efficient working practices, adequate communications, defined responsibilities and staff working within their competence.

Funding
- Identify resources. Can potential savings on medical and nursing time, or savings on drug expenditure be utilised?
- Is the hospital prepared to pay for increased safety and quality, and proactive risk management.
- Where does a CIVAS fit into a unit's priorities?

Personnel
- Are the funds available for appropriate levels of staff with the necessary level of expertise?
- Are funds available for recruitment and training?

Logistic points for consideration
- The physical geography of the site.
- Is more than one site being serviced?
- Communication and transport systems.
- Consultants' prescribing habits.

- Provision of first and 'stat' doses.
- Recovery and re-use.
- Distribution.
- Levels of service at weekends and holidays.
- Costing arrangements.
- On-call service versus a commitment to extended hours.
- Satellite facilities and staff.

Clinical commitment

The level of clinical involvement can be enhanced by providing a CIVAS. The level of patient care must be resourced and should not detract from the efficiency of the service and will depend on the attitudes of local personnel and their managers.

1.8 Is a Licence Required?

This will depend on the type of service, the nature and shelf-life of the products, the purchasers of the finished products and the range and size of the workload.

There are three types of manufacturer's licence:
- A manufacture and assembly licence covering the manufacture and assembly of medicinal products with product licences.
- An assembly only licence, restricted to the assembly only of medicinal products with product licences.
- A manufacturer's 'specials' licence.

As an exception to the need for a product licence, provision has been made for the manufacture of products as part of a 'special dispensing service' and allows the preparation of medicinal products in response to special orders received from retail pharmacists, hospitals, wholesalers and certain other persons or organisations.

A manufacturer's 'specials' licence is the type of licence appropriate to larger CIVAS. Alternatively, preparation for named patients may be carried out under an exemption conferred by section 10 of the *Medicines Act*.[4] It can also apply to preparing stock from which to dispense to named patients in accordance with a prescription provided that the conditions of the exemption are met.

- The preparation is done by or under the supervision of a pharmacist.
- The preparation uses closed systems.
- Licensed medicinal products are used as ingredients or the ingredients are manufactured in licensed facilities.

- Products are given an expiry date of no more than one week. The shelf-life should be supported by stability data.
- All activities should be in accordance with defined NHS guidelines.

1.9 Paediatric CIVAS

Most injections used for paediatric patients are available only as standard preparations reflecting the usual size of the adult dose. The great variation in weight and therefore dose requirement from birth to adolescence means that considerable wastage can occur when paediatric doses are withdrawn from 'adult size' vials and ampoules.

Some paediatric nurses and doctors will attempt to reduce wastage by re-using the injection solution from vials and ampoules. There is obviously potential for error, contamination, and loss of activity with this practice.

Wastage of intravenous drugs in a paediatric unit or hospital is likely to be in excess of 30% and provision of a paediatric CIVAS can make significant savings in drug expenditure in contrast to the much smaller savings (if any) achievable with injections for adults.

The presentation of intravenous additive doses in minibags for intermittent infusion to paediatric patients is usually inappropriate with fluid volumes being too large. Most intravenous additives for neonates and children should be presented in syringes for slow bolus administration, addition to a small volume of fluid in a burette administration set, or for administration using a syringe pump.

Standardisation of doses for adults allows preparation in advance and the holding of stocks at ward level. With the wide range of dose sizes required, this is unlikely to be possible in paediatric practice and will mean that a very responsive service must be provided to ensure accuracy of dosing with minimal wastage.

A similar situation is found on adult intensive care units where tailoring of drug dosage to weight, clinical condition and response is more likely than on general wards.

1.10 Use of an External Service

After having confirmed the need to provide an aseptically prepared product, pharmacy managers may consider using a service provided by a third party, either a commercial service or from an NHS unit. This may be done for a number of reasons, which may include the lack of appropriate facilities, space or available staff. The use of an external service may be considered as a temporary measure until these or other resources are obtained.

Before coming to a decision to use an external service there are a number of problems which need to be addressed.

The range and nature of external services
- Are external services available to meet all the needs for the provision of medication requiring aseptic preparation?

The nature of the products
The nature of some products and their presentation dictates that they must be prepared immediate to the site of use, therefore external preparation is not a viable option.

Management control of contracted services
The pharmacy manager has no control over processes since the pharmacy is the supplier of a purchased product rather than the provider of a service.

Cost effectiveness
Both the provision of an internal service and the purchase of an external service have to be carefully costed to include all factors which will determine the true cost of the prepared product. This will determine the cost effectiveness of the provision of either service.

Quality considerations
Quality must be the overriding concern when considering product or service options. Pharmacy managers must agree arrangements when purchasing

services, rather than have terms dictated by suppliers. It follows that measuring performance against quality control standards is a key issue.

A specification of service must be agreed and the specification document signed by the purchaser and provider. Appropriate licences, e.g. manufacturers 'specials' licence, should be held by the external provider.

Managers should be able to identify clear gains when purchasing aseptic compounding services. These should include the benefits that accrue from economies of scale. In addition, purchasing these services should free local resources including staff, capital and floor space to support other activities.

1.11 Use of a Satellite Service

The minimum standards acceptable in the aseptic preparation of parenteral products are those specified for 'good manufacturing practice'.[5] The standards for a satellite unit may differ, without any lowering of standards, from those which may be required locally for use in a centralised service.

1.12 References

1. Breckenridge A. HC(76)9: the report of the working party on the addition of drugs to intravenous fluids. London: Department of Health and Social Security, 1976.
2. Consumer protection act 1987. London: HMSO, 1987.
3. Farwell J. Aseptic dispensing for NHS patients. London: Department of Health, 1994.
4. Medicines Control Agency. Guidance to the NHS on the licensing requirements of the Medicines Act 1968. London: Medicines Control Agency, 1992.
5. Medicines Control Agency. Rules and guidance for pharmaceutical manufacturers and distributors 1997. London: The Stationery Office, 1997.

2 Costing a CIVAS

Christine Clarke and Christine Trehane

2.1 Introduction

There are two major components to be taken into consideration when costing a CIVAS, the overhead costs for running the unit, which may be part of a larger production department, and the specific cost of the batch or individual preparation. Some costs can be assigned accurately to a particular product, but others, such as the disposable tubing used for more than one patient specific preparation, or cleaning agents used for spraying isolators, can only be costed on a total yearly basis and apportioned according to the number of additives that are prepared annually. Exactly which costs are included will depend on the method chosen by the finance department within a particular hospital and the sophistication of the data retrieval systems in use.

2.2 Hospital Overheads

If the CIVAS does not stand alone, hospital costs for other services will have been costed for the whole hospital and a proportion of these allotted to the CIVAS. This allocation may be made on a floor area basis or as a proportion of the number of staff employed in the CIVAS against the hospital as a whole, or a mixture of the two may be used. Costs which come under this category may include:

- Trust senior management and administration.
- Cost of directorate management.
- Personnel and human resources.
- Cost of training courses run by the hospital.
- Office services.
- Domestic services (tendered and/or in-house).
- Security services.
- Fire service.
- Telephone service.
- Engineering department.
- Building and projects departments.
- General estate management.
- Energy, heating, water and sewage.
- Finance department.
- Supplies department.
- Occupational health department.
- Crèche facilities.

2.3 Departmental Overheads

The major component of departmental overheads is the cost of employing pharmacy staff who work directly or indirectly in the CIVAS. This includes all employer's costs, not just salaries and wages. If staff have other pharmacy duties, such as technician ward 'top-up', or ward pharmacy duties, the average time taken to carry out these duties should be estimated and the costs worked out on a pro-rata basis. The cost of running an in-house quality control service can be costed in a similar manner to production. Costs in this category include:

- Staff costs, including a proportion of the costs of porters, secretaries, buying officers, etc.
- Staff uniforms, white overalls and special aseptic clothing, including laundering and sterilisation.
- Cost of manufacturer's 'specials licence' (if applicable).
- Equipment (written off over a period of years).
- Equipment maintenance contracts.
- Specific facility upgrading.
- Staff travel and outside training courses.
- Items consumed, damaged, or rejected, which cannot be assigned to specific products.

2.4 Product Specific Costs

The total cost of all the items in the two above categories should be calculated and assigned, either on a time basis or divided between the total number of items prepared over a period of time to give an overhead. This may be weighted depending on the type of product produced. Product specific costs can be assigned as:

- Ingredient cost.
- Container cost.
- Overhead (as calculated above).
- Disposables, including syringes, tubing, etc. which can be assigned to a specific product.
- Quality control, including cost of pyrogen and sterility testing (if applicable).

The above costs should then be calculated in total and divided between the number of items actually released from quarantine for the specific batch to determine a unit cost.

3 Service Operation

Christine Trehane

3.1 Introduction

The operation of a CIVAS should be fully documented with standard operating procedures and worksheets; the following points should be considered.

3.2 Receipt of CIVAS Requests

Requests for an intravenous additive may be received from doctors, nurses, pharmacists, technicians, or outside agencies. The documentation accompanying a request for a preparation should be carefully considered and procedures established for processing requests, including those received via the telephone and fax. Usually, a paper copy of a CIVAS request should be obtained. Other electronic means of communication should also be considered such as via a hospital computer network.

3.3 Processing CIVAS Requests

It should be ensured that sufficient information is provided with a CIVAS request to check the drug dose and compliance with approved protocol, method of administration, and compatibility. A procedure for checking requests transmitted by means other than the original prescription should be established.

The method of administration, for example, syringe, infusion, elastomeric device, etc. should be confirmed. The standard concentration for reconstituting dry powder vials, suitable diluents, and the stability of the preparation should be considered. The dose should be calculated and checked.

The procedure for disposal of part-used vials or ampoules, and other 'sharps', such as needles, should also be established.

In many units, computer systems are used to process CIVAS requests, but a manual backup system should also be in place. Computer software should be validated.

3.4 CIVAS Documentation

It is essential that all procedures are thoroughly doc-umented and that complete records of all operations and preparations are maintained. Written procedures for the creation, review and up-dating of documents should be available and the procedures for copying master documents must be laid down. Documents, including written procedures and preparation records should be numbered and indexed, and appropriately stored in such a way that both current and archived documents are readily retrievable. Documentation should include:

- Personnel, training, and maintenance records.
- Quality assurance procedures and records.
- Patient and drug records (by ward and by drug).
- Data for workload statistics, stock control and costing.
- Financial and budgetary information.

The design of worksheets and labels should take account of all CIVAS batch production or dispensing activities. Worksheets for preparations stored frozen should allow for the freezing and thawing process and any re-labelling necessary.

Computer systems may be used to store and retrieve documents but a manual backup should also be available. Records must be stored for the statutory minimum period of time.

3.5 Drug Preparation

All staff involved in the preparation of intravenous additives should have successfully completed a suitable training course (*see* below) and be familiar with local operating procedures including the use of isolators, laminar flow cabinets (LFCs), and other equipment.

Procedures should be established for entering preparation areas (clean rooms) and changing into appropriate clothing. Consideration should also be given to the passing of drugs and equipment into and out of clean rooms, LFCs, and isolators.

The reconstitution and preparation method, including drug or dosage segregation, for a specific drug additive, should be considered and previously validated. The selection of preparation ingredients and equipment should also be considered. Checks should be made during additive preparation.

3.6 Labelling and Checking

Preparations should be carefully checked for any visual defects, and procedures followed for the generation of appropriate labels. Outer protective product wrapping should also be inspected.

A final check of the preparation, its packaging, labelling, and documentation should be made before the product is released for use.

3.7 Distribution and Storage

The storage of preparations, including frozen preparations, within a CIVAS should be considered. Storage conditions should be validated and monitored regularly.

The method of distribution of preparations within a hospital including the role of porters, nurses, and CIVAS staff should be considered. Procedures for the transportation of preparations off-site, for example to another hospital or to a 'home patient', must be established. Appropriate packaging should be used and attention given to the maintenance and validation of good storage practices, particularly for preparations which should be refrigerated. The role of drivers, other pharmacies, healthcare companies, district nurses, patients and their carers should be considered. Evidence of the maintenance of the 'cold chain' is important.

Procedures for the return of unused doses and for the destruction and disposal of 'out-of-date' material should be established.

3.8 Cleaning

Preparation areas should be regularly cleaned and disinfected in accordance with local procedures. Cleaning procedures should be documented and records kept.

Isolators and LFCs should be regularly cleaned and disinfected. Perishable parts, such as isolator gloves, should be routinely and frequently checked for wear and replaced when necessary. Isolators, LFCs, and other equipment should be regularly checked and maintained.

Local procedures for dealing with spillages, such as cleaning and decontamination, should be documented.

3.9 Quality Assurance

Intravenous additive units should operate an active quality assurance programme designed to check and validate procedures and staff.

Documentation, such as worksheets and procedures, should be regularly updated and checked. Operators, procedures, the working environment, and equipment, should initially be validated and thereafter regularly monitored. Records of validations and checks should be maintained. Containers and finished products should also be checked for sterility and drug content.

3.10 Training

An induction procedure should be followed for all grades of staff within a CIVAS. Staff should successfully complete a documented training programme before preparing any additives. Training programmes may involve 'broth tests' in which preparation procedures are followed using a growth medium which is indicative of microbiological contamination.

Staff should be trained in the use of computers and equipment and it should be established which staff are authorised to carry out, or check, particular processes or operations.

Staff should be regularly re-trained and checked and a record of training kept. This topic is referred to in more detail in chapter 4.

3.11 Stock Control

Good stock control is essential for the economic and efficient operation of a CIVAS. Adequate quantities of drugs and raw materials should be maintained and stock rotated to ensure the minimum of wastage due to 'out-of-date' stock.

Stock should be stored in an appropriate location and its receipt, batch number, and expiry date, documented. Systems for returning expired stock and still usable products, and methods for the re-cycling of doses (if appropriate) should be established.

3.12 Computers

Extensive use of computer systems can be made to ensure the efficient operation of a CIVAS. Various CIVAS, total parenteral nutrition (TPN) and cytotoxic programs are available which may be used to produce worksheets and labels, and to store preparation and training documentation.

CIVAS computer systems may also be usefully connected to a main pharmacy department system or to other networks within a hospital such as the finance department, or to prescribing systems.

Any computer programs used should be validated and manual backup systems established.

Consideration must be given to the retrieval of any archive material when the software or hardware currently in use is superseded.

4 CIVAS Training

James Thom

4.1 Introduction

Training needs are linked to the level of understanding required for the various roles involved in providing an effective and efficient service.

At one end of this spectrum will be the training requirements for operatives involved in producing medium to large scale batches of routine preparations. Towards the other end are the training needs of those individuals involved in planning and managing a CIVAS. In the latter group, training is usually part of the continuing professional education process and may involve project work or even original research.

4.2 Operative Training

In general, operatives can be divided into three groups:

- Those performing well-defined and tightly controlled routine processes under constant direct, or indirect supervision where the level of understanding required is relatively low, such as batch production, where materials are accounted for going in and out of the processing stage.
- Those performing well-defined and controlled processes with a low level of direct supervision, and where the level of understanding required is low to moderate.
- Those involved in setting up services from scratch, expanding into new areas, and developing processes and procedures new to the unit.

Obviously, the number of operatives and their grades will be dependent on workload and funding. Where there is a low to moderate workload, staff segregation and stratification may not be appropriate. However, it is common for CIVAS demand to grow exponentially and managers should bear this in mind when planning for staff recruitment, training, and equipment.

Most operative training for the first group will be practically orientated and performed on a one-to-one basis. A checklist of all the areas of training covered, signed by the trainee, supervisor, and assessor,

can form a useful guide and personal record of progress. This should include performance indicators such as:

- Broth transfer test results.
- Averaged finger-dab culture records.
- Standard solution transfer results.
- Accident records (e.g. needle-stick injuries).

Checklists can be used for staff training in aseptic work at all levels, e.g. unqualified staff and student technicians (Group 1). In this group, a high level of initial training and re-training and monitoring is required as the workforce is unskilled. This group may take a disproportionate amount of time to train as they usually have little or no relevant previous experience.

Preregistration pharmacy graduates and technicians form Group 2, where less 'training' is required as they should have acquired the basics in their previous studies and training.

Senior technicians and pharmacist managers form Group 3, and may require different skills, such as management, and research and development skills. These may be acquired 'in-house' but may also necessitate study days or courses where applicable.

The latter group may be the most costly in terms of capital outlay if skills are not available at the base hospital.

The checklists have been designed to allow gradual and methodical training, and recording of such training, to be given to the trainee. It is important that adequate records of training are kept so that the individual competency is known and assessed regularly. The checklists can be used to point out areas of re-training that are required.

Checklists have been developed for the following areas (*see* section 4.4):

- Aseptic introduction.
- Batched CIVAS/TPN.
- Individual CIVAS/TPN.
- Batched and individual cytotoxics.
- Quality assurance/control awareness.

The aseptic introduction is designed to develop an

awareness of:

- Terminology and abbreviations.
- General principles of aseptic technique, facilities and equipment.
- Materials and methods involved.
- Patients and clinical areas served.

The batched CIVAS/TPN checklist is targeted towards the training needs of Group 1 type operators and covers:

- Terminology and equipment specific to these procedures.
- The individuals' understanding of the general and specific processes and procedures involved.
- The practice assessments and results of broth transfers, settle, and finger-dab plates and initial participation in batched CIVAS/TPN.

The individual CIVAS/TPN check list is targeted towards Group 2 and 3 operatives and covers:

- Patients, prescriptions and relevant clinical data.
- Drug/product information especially on stability/compatibility.
- Methodologies.
- Techniques.
- Procedures.
- Practice assessments.

4.3 Management Training/Research and Development Programme

Management training falls somewhat outside the scope of this review although the management approach tends to dictate the recruitment policy and thus, in turn, basic training requirements. Where the emphasis is on cytotoxic and tailored CIVAS/TPN production the level of expertise required may be such that experienced, well-trained staff need to be recruited from outside the organisation. Once these services are established the service can expand to cover batched production of 'stock' CIVAS/TPN. Operatives for this area are probably best recruited from the existing staff, where suitable candidates exist. This has certainly been the approach used by successful companies who select CIVAS/TPN production staff from well-established staff members.

As CIVAS is an area of rapid growth in terms of demand, workload, and knowledge, it is important that senior management (who carry overall responsibility) are fully aware of and are able to control and plan future developments. Methods for accomplishing this are:

- Study day attendances and self-development training.
- Visits to centres of 'excellence'.
- Peer group reviews.
- Encouraging a climate of challenge and change.
- Encouraging projects in relevant areas of practice research.
- Actively participating in providing/reviewing performance and quality initiatives.
- Business planning.
- Internal and external audit.

4.4 Technical Services Training Checklists

The following checklists are provided as guidance and may be adapted for individual needs.

Aseptic Introduction 1

Name:		Start:	Finish:
Subject/Task	**Date**	**Trainee**	**Trainer**
Terminology and Abbreviations			
TPN/CIVAS/cytotoxics/QC/QA			
SCBU/ICU/HEPA/HLF/VLF/COSHH/H&S			
MCA/Occupational Health Dept./mL/mmol/mg/mcg/%			
BP/BPC/BNF/HF			
Aseptic Facilities			
Suite/change-double-three level			
Interlock/communications/intercoms/pass through hatches			
Laminar airflow/product protection/isolators			
Operator protection/clean room protective garments			
Hoods/boots/gloves/double gloving			
Equipment			
Ampoules and snapules/bags and minibags/bottles/vials/ports			
Venting devices/spikes/needles			
Filters and filter needles/filling tubes/syringes/luer fittings			
Caps/closures/leads/transfer sets			
Connectors/pumps-drivers (automated and peristaltic)/computers			
Aseptic Technique			
Rationale/cabinet working			
Hygiene rules/changing procedures			
Open and closed procedures/reconstitution/aspiration			
Aerosol/air bubbles/particulate contamination			
Hazard prevention and removal			
Validation			
Monitoring/waste disposal and sharps			

Assessed by: Date: Comments:

Aseptic Introduction 2

Name:		Start:	Finish:
Subject/Task	Date	Trainee	Trainer
Materials			
Lyophilised powders/emulsions/solutions			
Colloids and suspensions/antibiotics			
Cytotoxics/nutrients/tests/solutions			
Methods			
Procedures: general and specific (awareness)			
Worksheets/labels/calculations/checks/packaging/despatch			
QC/assays/tests/controls			
QA/environmental monitoring/health checks			
Patients			
Immunocompromised/chemotherapy/renal			
Intensive care/neurology/neurosurgery			
Neonates/paediatrics/rheumatology/special			
Other			
Fire and evacuation procedure			
Health and safety			
Accident policy			

Assessed by: Date: Comments:

Batched CIVAS/TPN

Name:		Start:	Finish:
Subject/Task	Date	Trainee	Trainer
Terminology and Equipment			
TPN: amino acid solutions/fat emulsions/glucose			
TPN: vitamins/trace elements/electrolytes/EVA bags			
TPN: compounding devices/specific gravity/calibrations			
TPN: leads/filling/capping and sealing/giving sets			
CIVAS: minibags/tamper proofing/fluids			
CIVAS: dispensing/semi-automatic syringe filling/elastomeric devices			
CIVAS: syringe capping/heat sealing			
Procedures (has read and understood)			
Changing procedure			
Procedure for use of the compounding device			
General CIVAS preparation procedures			
Batched CIVAS/TPN procedure			
CIVAS/TPN costing procedure			
Process COSHH assessments			
Settle plate monitoring procedure and finger-dab plate procedure			
Broth transfer procedures (CIVAS and TPN)			
Practice (has satisfactorily carried out)			
TPN broth transfer			
CIVAS syringe broth transfer			
Finger-dab plate procedure/settle plate exposure			
Participation in batch TPN production			
Participation in batch CIVAS production			
Techniques			
Syringe use/ampoule opening/drawing up			
Venting/air bubble prevention and removal			
Aerosol formation prevention and control			
Compounding device/programming/gravity feed filling			
Volumetric/vacuum filling			

Assessed by: Date: Comments:

Individual CIVAS/TPN

Name:			Start:	Finish:
Subject/Task		**Date**	**Trainee**	**Trainer**
Patients and Prescriptions (wards, ward pharmacists, and technicians)				
Liaison/telephoned, faxed, and computer-generated orders				
Dose/protocol/frequency/length of treatment/checks				
Files/records and receipt of orders				
Routes of administration/drug delivery techniques				
Bolus IV/IV infusion/IM/IT/SC				
Central and peripheral lines				
Syringe pumps/drivers in use/PCA/portable devices				
Clinical Data				
Administration procedures/protocols/schedules				
Laboratory tests and monitoring/adverse reactions				
Extravasation/pharmacokinetic introduction/adverse reactions				
Drug and Product Information				
Compatibility/incompatibility/interactions				
Stability/data sheets/local 'other'				
Osmolarity and pH/displacement values				
Methods				
Calculations/fractions/decimals/percentages/proportions				
Units and conversions				
Computers/compounding machine programme				
Manufacturing programme/CIVAS and TPN programme				
Label requirements/label and worksheet generation				

Assessed by: Date: Comments:

Quality Assurance Awareness

Name:		Start:	Finish:
Subject/Task	Date	Trainee	Trainer
Terminology			
Quality control/quality assurance			
Stability/shelf-life			
Storage			
Analysis			
Assay/electrolyte levels			
Refractive index/UV spectrophotometry/visual			
Sterility testing			
Broth transfers (CIVAS and TPN)			
Safety and accuracy assessment (quinine sulphate)			
Finger-dab plates/settle plates/surface swabs/contact plates			
Environment			
Classification/class E/F (as EC GMP)			
Class J and K (C and D, EC GMP)			
Environmental monitoring			
Over-pressures/pressure drop indicator			
Temperature/relative humidity/particle counts			
Microbiological monitoring (active and passive)			
Airflow rates and patterns			
Sampling			
Random sampling			
Uniform sample withdrawal			

Assessed by: Date: Comments:

Practice Results/Assessment

Name:...

	Date	Result	Date	Result
Broth transfer: TPN				
Broth transfer: CIVAS (syringes)				
	Period	**Result**	**Period**	**Result**
Finger-dab plate (averaged)				
Settle plate screen (averaged)				
Settle plate change (averaged)				
Batch TPN (averaged)				
Batch CIVAS (averaged)				

Assessed by: Date: Comments:

Signed:...   Trainee

Signed:...   Trainer

Signed:...   Assessor

Review Date:...

5 Quality Assurance Audit of a CIVAS

Mike Booth

5.1 Introduction

This section aims to set the broad framework for an audit to be conducted on intravenous additive services prepared in hospital pharmacies. Standards quoted comply with good manufacturing practice (GMP) and good dispensing practice (GDP) along with other statutory requirements. It is intended as a guide to the questions that should be asked during an audit. However, not all units will have the facilities described, e.g. both laminar flow cabinets (LFCs) and isolators, and this should be taken into account when devising local audit documents.

5.2 Guidance Notes

Audit results should be graded according to a number '1–4' which represents compliance or non-compliance according to the following criteria:

1. Critical non-compliance (manufacturing activities should stop and immediate remedial action should be taken)
2. Major non-compliance
3. Minor non-compliance
4. Compliance with acceptance criteria

N/A Not applicable

5.3 Audit Worksheets

Table 1: Policies and standards

Table 2: Facilities and premises

Table 3: Equipment

Table 4: Environmental acceptability

Table 5: Operator protection

Table 6: Procedures, documentation, and formulation

Table 7: Compounding and preparation

Table 8: Labelling and presentation

Table 9: Quality assurance and audit

Table 10: Storage, distribution, and administration

Table 11: Personnel and training

Table 12: Health and safety

Table 13: Effective use of resources

Table 14: Handling of complaints and anomalies

Table 15: Product shelf-life

Table 1: Policies and standards

No.	Acceptance criteria	Check required	Audit result	Comments/ Action
1.1	Standards of dispensing and preparation of stock should be identified and where appropriate considered the same.	Assess	1 2 3 4 N/A	
1.2	Guidance documents to be applied are: Lee MG, Midcalf B, editors. Isolators for pharmaceutical applications. London: HMSO, 1994. Medicines Control Agency. Guidance to the NHS on the licensing requirements of the Medicines Act 1968. London: Medicines Control Agency, 1992. Medicines Control Agency. Rules and guidance for pharmaceutical manufacturers. London: The Stationery Office, 1997. Needle R, Sizer T, editors. CIVAS handbook. London: Pharmaceutical Press, 1998. NHS Quality Control Committee. The quality assurance of aseptic preparation services, 2nd edition. London: HMSO, 1996. Royal Pharmaceutical Society. Medicines, ethics and practice: a guide for pharmacists 19. London: Royal Pharmaceutical Society, 1998.	Assess	1 2 3 4 N/A	
1.3	General policy statement published including principles of services, premises, and review date.	Examine	1 2 3 4 N/A	
1.4	Processes and procedures must be designed, validated, and documented. If deviations occur, these must be controlled, audited, and documented.	Assess	1 2 3 4 N/A	
1.5	Status of unit checked for compliance with legal standards i.e. licensed or unlicensed.	Assess	1 2 3 4 N/A	
1.6	All processes to be carried out must be assessed and validated by the responsible pharmacist before processes are put into operation.	Examine	1 2 3 4 N/A	
1.7	Any deviations from validated processes must be recorded and assessed by the responsible pharmacist.	Examine	1 2 3 4 N/A	

Table 2: Facilities and premises

No.	Acceptance criteria	Check required	Audit result	Comments/ Action
2.1	Facilities are of an adequate size for the activities undertaken.	Assess	1 2 3 4 N/A	
2.2	Facilities incorporate appropriate design features in terms of current GMP, ergonomics and work flow, e.g. clean room design.	Assess	1 2 3 4 N/A	
2.3	Walls, floors, ceilings, and work surfaces are cleaned according to validated procedures.	Examine	1 2 3 4 N/A	
2.4	Facilities are in good decorative order and are maintained to an appropriate standard.	Assess	1 2 3 4 N/A	
2.5	Operation, cleaning, maintenance, and fault logs kept up to date.	Examine	1 2 3 4 N/A	
2.6	Cleaning procedures are regularly validated particularly when hazardous material is present.	Examine	1 2 3 4 N/A	

Table 3: Equipment

No.	Acceptance criteria	Check required	Audit result	Comments/ Action
3.1	Equipment is appropriate for the operational procedures undertaken.	Assess	1 2 3 4 N/A	
3.2	Equipment is serviced and maintained at appropriate specified intervals and records kept.	Records	1 2 3 4 N/A	
3.3	Operational characteristics of key equipment are confirmed in writing as part of planned preventative maintenance.	Assess	1 2 3 4 N/A	
3.4	Written operating procedures are available for all equipment.	Procedure	1 2 3 4 N/A	
3.5	Where appropriate, equipment is tested against performance criteria for compliance with appropriate guidelines and standards (e.g. HTM10, GMP, regional policies).	Assess	1 2 3 4 N/A	
3.6	Equipment is kept clean and protected from unnecessary damage, heat and dust.	Observe	1 2 3 4 N/A	

Table 4: Environmental acceptability

No.	Acceptance criteria	Check required	Audit result	Comments/Action
	Rooms and laminar flow cabinets			
4.1	Room(s) design, condition, and repair complies with the general requirements of BS 5295 (1989).	Assess	1 2 3 4 N/A	
4.2	Room(s) comply with grade B (unmanned) air and are tested every month.	Records	1 2 3 4 N/A	
4.3	Room(s) comply with the relevant local standards for filter leak tests, manometer readings, active air sampling, airflow direction and air change measurements, airflow patterns and pressure differentials.	Records	1 2 3 4 N/A	
4.4	Laminar flow cabinet complies with grade A (unmanned) air and is tested every month.	Records	1 2 3 4 N/A	
4.5	Laminar flow cabinet complies with BS 5726 for air velocity, direction, and safety requirements.	Records	1 2 3 4 N/A	
4.6	Laminar flow cabinet complies with KI test and is tested every 13 months.	Records	1 2 3 4 N/A	
4.7	Procedures reflect current standards of aseptic practice and technique.	Observe/Procedure	1 2 3 4 N/A	
4.8	Both the room(s) and the laminar flow cabinet comply with the local standards for acceptable levels of micro-organisms, e.g. settle plates, and are tested weekly. Limits must be set. Sessional plates must be used.	Records	1 2 3 4 N/A	
4.9	Operators must comply with standards set for acceptable levels of micro-organisms, e.g. finger dabs, and must be tested weekly. Limits must be set.	Records	1 2 3 4 N/A	
4.10	Limits exceeded have documented action taken.	Examine	1 2 3 4 N/A	
4.11	Appropriate records kept of environmental monitoring.	Records	1 2 3 4 N/A	
4.12	Cleaning records comply with written schedules.	Records	1 2 3 4 N/A	
	Isolators			
4.13	Both the room(s) and the isolator comply with the local standards for acceptable levels of micro-organisms, e.g. settle plates, and are tested weekly. Limits must be set. Sessional plates must be used.	Records	1 2 3 4 N/A	
4.14	Isolators(s) should be sited in a dedicated area, with an appropriate background air quality.	Assess	1 2 3 4 N/A	
4.15	The controlled workspace, critical zone and transfer device of the isolator complies with grade A (unmanned).	Records	1 2 3 4 N/A	
4.16	Monitoring of the isolator and the room complies with standards laid down in *Isolators for Pharmaceutical Applications*.	Records	1 2 3 4 N/A	
4.17	Gloves and gauntlets used with the isolator comply with the limits for perforations specified in BS 4005.	Records	1 2 3 4 N/A	

Table 5: Operator protection

No.	Acceptance criteria	Check required	Audit result	Comments/ Action
5.1	Appropriate type of clothing, including masks and gloves, to locally accepted standard.	Assess	1 2 3 4 N/A	
5.2	Clothing cleaned appropriately and monitored.	Assess	1 2 3 4 N/A	
5.3	Clothing, including gloves, changed at designated intervals.	Assess	1 2 3 4 N/A	
5.4	Venting filter or aspiration systems used to prevent positive pressure within vials.	Observe/Procedure	1 2 3 4 N/A	
5.5	Validated procedure for dealing with spillages in place, e.g. cytotoxics or penicillins.	Procedure	1 2 3 4 N/A	
5.6	Appropriate disposal of consumables including vials, syringes and needles.	Procedure/Assess	1 2 3 4 N/A	
5.7	Procedure for disposal of contained waste with reference to COSHH regulations 1989.	Procedure/Assess	1 2 3 4 N/A	

Table 6: Procedures, documentation, and formulation

No.	Acceptance criteria	Check required	Audit result	Comments/ Action
6.1	Standard operating procedures written for all processes and equipment and issued, approved, and reviewed by suitably qualified staff. Key areas: • changing procedures • cleaning procedures • maintenance and servicing of equipment, premises • environmental and microbiological control • quality control and quality assurance • health and safety policy including COSHH	Examine Examine Examine Examine Examine Examine	1 2 3 4 N/A 1 2 3 4 N/A 1 2 3 4 N/A 1 2 3 4 N/A 1 2 3 4 N/A 1 2 3 4 N/A	
6.2	Control system established to ensure only up-to-date documentation and programmes used.	Examine	1 2 3 4 N/A	
6.3	Master batch manufacturing records formulae/worksheets written and approved by suitably qualified staff.	Examine	1 2 3 4 N/A	
6.4	Formulations have been validated for stability (published or in-house evidence).	Examine	1 2 3 4 N/A	
6.5	Formulations and documentation are approved by suitably qualified staff.	Examine	1 2 3 4 N/A	
6.6	Stability, compatibility, and expiry, checked and approved by suitably qualified staff.	Examine	1 2 3 4 N/A	
6.7	A formal procedure for notifying appropriate staff when a fault, defect, problem or other exception arises. The notification is in writing and when completed describes the exception, the action taken, and by whom, and the outcome.	Examine	1 2 3 4 N/A	
6.8	Computer software programs are validated initially, after alteration or transfer to a separate machine, and documented.	Examine	1 2 3 4 N/A	

Table 7: Compounding and preparation

No.	Acceptance criteria	Check required	Audit result	Comments/ Action
7.1	Critical stages of the process must be identified, e.g. preparation and filling.	Examine	1 2 3 4 N/A	
7.2	Materials, devices, and containers must be from approved suppliers only.	Records	1 2 3 4 N/A	
7.3	Documentary evidence of correct reconstitution.	Records	1 2 3 4 N/A	
7.4	Documents satisfactorily completed.	Records	1 2 3 4 N/A	
7.5	Check each drug is correctly incorporated into the appropriate syringe/bag.	Examine	1 2 3 4 N/A	
7.6	Filter integrity test is satisfactory for each filter used (if appropriate).	Observe	1 2 3 4 N/A	
7.7	Appropriate segregation techniques are employed if different product types share common facilities.	Examine	1 2 3 4 N/A	
7.8	All preparations are clear and free from visible particles.	Examine	1 2 3 4 N/A	
7.9	Operators must have their eye-sight checked and recorded.	Examine	1 2 3 4 N/A	

Table 8: Labelling and presentation

No.	Acceptance criteria	Check required	Audit result	Comments/ Action
8.1	Label is unambiguous, legible, and bears all relevant information, i.e. patient's name, ingredients, storage conditions, expiry date, and precautionary labels.	Examine	1 2 3 4 N/A	
8.2	Labels should be approved, controlled, and reconciled by appropriately qualified staff.	Assess	1 2 3 4 N/A	
8.3	Outer packaging is approved, appropriate, and secure.	Examine	1 2 3 4 N/A	
8.4	Product requires minimal manipulation at point of use.	Assess	1 2 3 4 N/A	
8.5	Each container checked for integrity and intactness.	Examine	1 2 3 4 N/A	
8.6	Syringes must be of the luer lock type and sealed with appropriate cap.	Examine	1 2 3 4 N/A	
8.7	Each syringe checked for fill volume and absence of air bubbles.	Examine	1 2 3 4 N/A	
8.8	Containers of clear plastic unless light protection necessary.	Examine	1 2 3 4 N/A	

Table 9: Quality assurance and audit

No.	Acceptance criteria	Check required	Audit result	Comments/ Action
9.1	A comprehensive quality assurance programme is set up by the responsible pharmacist and quality controller.	Assess	1 2 3 4 N/A	
9.2	Raw material specifications written e.g. container specifications.	Examine	1 2 3 4 N/A	
9.3	Microbiological testing (minimum weekly) performed on random samples of any unused product, and specially prepared samples. Note, not cytotoxic samples.	Records	1 2 3 4 N/A	
9.4	Unused product tested against finished product specifications.	Records	1 2 3 4 N/A	
9.5	Check and release procedures controlled by a suitably qualified and authorised pharmacist.	Assess	1 2 3 4 N/A	
9.6	Independent suitably trained and experienced staff conduct the audit.	Assess	1 2 3 4 N/A	
9.7	System of controls in place to establish fault/remedial action plans.	Records	1 2 3 4 N/A	
9.8	Regular review of the quality assurance programme undertaken.	Examine	1 2 3 4 N/A	

Table 10: Storage, distribution, and administration

No.	Acceptance criteria	Check required	Audit result	Comments/ Action
10.1	Syringe/bag suitably protected for transport to ward e.g. hermetically-sealed plastic (tamper evident) bags and in transport bags or similar to protect against heat, light, and physical damage.	Examine	1 2 3 4 N/A	
10.2	Storage in the pharmacy is validated and routinely monitored e.g. refrigeration.	Records	1 2 3 4 N/A	
10.3	Storage on the wards is validated and routinely monitored.	Records	1 2 3 4 N/A	
10.4	Delivery system to wards ensures patient receives syringe/bag at correct time.	Records	1 2 3 4 N/A	
10.5	Returned product must have a known history and a vaild shelf-life, and be assessed for re-use by a suitably qualified person.	Records	1 2 3 4 N/A	
10.6	Returned product must be via a validated cold chain.	Examine	1 2 3 4 N/A	

Table 11: Personnel and training

No.	Acceptance criteria	Check required	Audit result	Comments/ Action
11.1	An agreed and defined management structure including a named 'responsible pharmacist'.	Examine	1 2 3 4 N/A	
11.2	Sufficient appropriately trained, qualified staff available for the needs of the service.	Assess	1 2 3 4 N/A	
11.3	Written training and education manual.	Examine	1 2 3 4 N/A	
11.4	Staff perform satisfactory broth transfers or approved local test method at defined regular intervals e.g. six monthly.	Records	1 2 3 4 N/A	
11.5	Process should be validated using broth transfers or approved local test method at defined intervals e.g. six monthly.	Records	1 2 3 4 N/A	
11.6	Health screening and monitoring carried out if appropriate especially where personal circumstances change i.e. becoming pregnant.	Assess	1 2 3 4 N/A	
11.7	Engineers and other service personnel should be suitably trained in the nature of the work.	Assess	1 2 3 4 N/A	
11.8	Records of continuing staff training.	Examine	1 2 3 4 N/A	

Table 12: Health and safety

No.	Acceptance criteria	Check required	Audit result	Comments/ Action
12.1	CIVAS health and safety policy written.	Examine	1 2 3 4 N/A	
12.2	COSHH assessments carried out on all commonly used products.	Assess	1 2 3 4 N/A	
12.3	Staff training manual incorporates health and safety legal requirements.	Assess	1 2 3 4 N/A	
12.4	Accident report book available.	Records	1 2 3 4 N/A	
12.5	Other hospital staff e.g. nurses and porters are aware of problems and spillage kits are available.	Assess	1 2 3 4 N/A	

Table 13: Effective use of resources

No.	Acceptance criteria	Check required	Audit result	Comments/ Action
13.1	Planned scheduling of workload.	Assess	1 2 3 4 N/A	
13.2	Minimise waste by choice of drug strengths, pack size, etc.	Assess	1 2 3 4 N/A	
13.3	Economic purchase of raw materials, consumables, etc.	Assess	1 2 3 4 N/A	
13.4	Use of approved suppliers of contracted support services.	Assess	1 2 3 4 N/A	

Table 14: Handling of complaints and anomalies

No.	Acceptance criteria	Check required	Audit result	Comments/ Action
14.1	All complaints recorded in the log book.	Assess	1 2 3 4 N/A	
14.2	All complaints investigated promptly and effectively to prevent recurrence.	Records	1 2 3 4 N/A	

Table 15: Product shelf-life

No.	Acceptance criteria	Check required	Audit result	Comments/ Action
15.1	Maximum shelf-life of seven days if no chemical or physical reasons for less. (Unlicensed units.)	Examine	1 2 3 4 N/A	
15.2	Shelf-life validated locally from all reliable sources of information.	Assess	1 2 3 4 N/A	

6 Selected Bibliography

Steve Brown

6.1 Aseptic Dispensing (General)

Chief Administrative Pharmaceutical Officers Committee. Standards for pharmaceutical care in health board premises and NHS trusts in Scotland, 1992.

Chief Administrative Pharmaceutical Officers Committee. Standards for pharmaceutical services in provider units in Wales, 1993.

Directors of Pharmaceutical Services of H&SS Boards (N. Ireland). Monitoring the quality of pharmaceutical services in NHS trusts/DMUs, 1993.

Farwell J. Aseptic dispensing for NHS patients. London: Department of Health, 1994.

Lund W, editor. The pharmaceutical codex: principles and practice of pharmaceutics, 12th edition. London: The Pharmaceutical Press, 1994.

Medicines Control Agency. Guidance to the NHS on the licensing requirements of the medicines act 1968. London: Medicines Control Agency, 1992.

Medicines Control Agency. Rules and guidance for pharmaceutical manufacturers. London: HMSO, 1993.

Medicines Control Agency. Rules and guidance for pharmaceutical manufacturers and distributors 1997. London: The Stationery Office, 1997.

NHS Quality Control Committee. The quality assurance of aseptic preparation services, 2nd edition. London: HMSO, 1996.

Regional Pharmaceutical Officers' Special Interest Group. Standards for pharmaceutical services in health authorities, units and trusts in England, 1991.

Regional Quality Control Subcommittee of the Regional Pharmaceutical Officers. Unlicensed medicines: notes for prescribers and pharmacists, 1993.

6.2 Aseptic Dispensing (Equipment)

British Standards Institute. Microbiological safety cabinets (BS 5276: parts 1,2,3,4). London: British Standards Institute, 1992.

Lee GM, Midcalf B, editors. Isolators for pharmaceutical applications. London: HMSO, 1994.

6.3 Aseptic Dispensing (Environment)

British Standards Institute. Environmental cleanliness in enclosed spaces (BS 5295: parts 0,1,2,3,4). London: British Standards Institute, 1989.

NHS Quality Control Committee. Detection methods for chemical contaminants. London: Department of Health, 1996.

Parenteral Society. Environmental contamination control practice, technical monograph No. 2. Swindon: Parenteral Society, 1989.

6.4 CIVAS Stability

Baker B. Aspects of product stability in central intravenous additive services. Hosp Pharm 1997; 4: 37-8.

Trissel LA. Handbook on injectable drugs, 9th edition. Bethesda, MD: American Society of Health-System Pharmacists Inc, 1996.

6.5 Intravenous Administration

Allwood M. Drug stability and intravenous administration: clinical pharmacy practice guide No. 14, 2nd edition. United Kingdom Clinical Pharmacy Association, 1994.

Medical Devices Agency. Device bulletin: infusion systems (MDA DB 9503). London: Medical Devices Agency, 1995.

Sani MH. Guide to intravenous drug therapy administration, 2nd edition. London: Guy's Hospital, 1996.

Scottish Office Home and Health Department. The management of infusion systems. London: Department of Health, 1995.

6.6 Other Useful References

Allwood M, Stanley A, Wright P, editors. The cytotoxics handbook, 3rd edition. Oxford: Radcliffe Medical Press, 1997.

Breckenridge A. HC(76)9: report of the working party on the addition of drugs to intravenous infusion fluids. London: Department of Helath and Social Security, 1976.

Needle R. The feasibility of centralised intravenous additive services. Hosp Pharm 1997; 4: 33-6.

Parenteral Drug Association. Validation of aseptic filling for solution drug products, technical monograph No. 2. Parenteral Drug Association (USA), 1987.

Sharp J. Good manufacturing practice: philosophy and applications. Buffalo Grove, IL: Interpharm Press, 1991.

Sharp J. Quality rules in sterile products manufacture. Woodley, Berkshire: John Sharp, 1992.

Draft technical assistance bulletin on quality assurance for pharmacy-prepared sterile products. Am J Hosp Pharm 1993; 50: 1440-52.

7 Stability of CIVAS Preparations

Brian Baker and Frank Haines-Nutt

7.1 Introduction

The growth in CIVAS has been limited by two major problems; the lack of suitable data for centrally prepared injections and the *British Pharmacopoeia* recommendation that unpreserved injections prepared aseptically from sterile ingredients should have a shelf-life of no greater than 24 hours. The licensing authorities have also tended to put a blanket restriction of a maximum of 24 hours on the shelf-life for reconstituted injectables.

The overriding reason for a 24 hour shelf-life for reconstituted injections is the risk of microbiological contamination of the product during preparation, reconstitution, or storage. The Medicines Control Agency (MCA) in their document *Guidance to the NHS on the Licensing Requirements of the Medicines Act*,[1] published in September 1992, have accepted that for unlicensed premises, products may be given an expiry date of up to one week, provided that the shelf-life is supported by stability data, the preparation is done by or under the supervision of a pharmacist using closed systems, and that licensed medicinal products or ingredients, manufactured in licensed facilities, are used. All activities must also be in accordance with defined NHS guidelines which were first published in January 1993 by the Quality Control Subcommittee of the Regional Pharmaceutical Officers and have been further reinforced by the publication *Aseptic Dispensing for NHS Patients*,[2] published by the Department of Health in England and Northern Ireland, and by the Welsh and Scottish Offices in December 1994. This document is commonly referred to as the *Farwell Document*.

The aseptic preparation facilities in many hospitals now comply with the above documents and enable the preparation of injections in controlled and validated environments where an acceptable level of sterility assurance and testing can be applied. Under these circumstances, the expiry date allocated should give equal weight to both the chemical properties of the preparation and the microbiological integrity of the process. If aseptic dispensing takes place in facilities which do not comply with these guidelines or is undertaken on the ward by medical or nursing staff, then the dispensed item should be used immediately and certainly should have a shelf-life of no greater than 24 hours.

The *Farwell Document* states that stability data available from manufacturers' official compendia or other reliable sources may be used, but must be carefully and reliably compared to ensure that the transfer to the local situation is justified. The following notes are intended to give general guidance when using these sources.

The report of the Regional Quality Control Subcommittee of the Regional Pharmaceutical Officers, published in the *Pharmaceutical Journal*,[3] pointed out that, in general, leaching from plastic syringes and bags is not a problem. However, sorption to, or incompatibility with, the plastic (as well as the physical and chemical stabilities of the solutions) still needs to be assessed. For example, etoposide was found to be totally incompatible with Sabre syringes, but initially compatible with polypropylene syringes.[4] Similarly, when methotrexate was stored in syringes with blind hubs, there was no sign of degradation after six weeks, but when stored in syringes fitted with needles precipitation occurred within 24 hours. The amsacrine solvent, dimethylacetamide, did not leach anything from two-piece polypropylene syringes over three days, but did from three-piece syringes which have a rubber plunger. The increasing use of lipid solutions in CIVAS will necessitate examination of these solutions in all available syringes.

To increase the assurance of microbial patency, reconstituted injections are usually kept in a refrigerator, and this normally also increases the shelf-life. However, there are examples where the concentrations required in a syringe are such that precipitation may occur in a refrigerator (e.g. aciclovir).[5] Ampicillin and cephradine are also less stable at higher than at lower concentrations. In the case of ampicillin, this is caused by polymerisation following collisions between molecules at the higher concentrations, with hydrolysis becoming the dominant degradation pathway at lower concentrations.[6,7]

It can be seen that it is very important to be cautious when assessing data derived from the literature, and to ensure that similar systems and concentrations are being used to those described in the reference. It is also possible to have apparent discrepancies between published shelf-lives, even with similar formulations, containers, and storage conditions. For example, one report might assign a shelf-life of 72 hours to a product, while another might give an identical product two weeks. In cases like this it is essential to know what questions were asked originally for an accurate interpretation to be put on the results. If a unit asks, 'Is a product stable for three days?' then it is possible for the laboratory to test for five days to obtain the required answer, whereas if the question asked is, 'How stable is the product?' then a longer testing period will be used, thus producing the longer shelf-life. It is advisable, therefore, to consult the original article or author.

Data and information may be derived from various sources including:

- Drug manufacturers.
- UK Regional Quality Controllers' Subcommittee.
- UK Stability Database (Contact: Dr P Grassby, Pharmaceutical Unit, St Mary's Hospital, Penarth).
- Pharmaceutical organisations.
- Various publications (*see* chapter 6).

On receiving a request for a preparation that has not previously been prepared within a CIVAS, the following action should be taken:

- Consult section 7.3 for appropriate references.
- Critically consider all the relevant primary references.
- Consider the final drug presentation required, the available storage conditions, and the length of shelf-life required.
- Consider the available preparation facilities, and the production method.

- Consider risk factors such as sterility assurance, use and administration (e.g. intrathecal), and transportation.
- Taking all of the above points into consideration assign a shelf-life.
- Reconfirm shelf-life by stability studies or by reference to comparable published studies.

The stability data in section 7.3 have been compiled over a number of years by one of the authors (Frank Haines-Nutt). The initial intention was to supplement the available US publications with information published in Europe. Practically all the information has been gathered from primary reference sources although, where appropriate for completeness, information from secondary sources has also been included.

Some references contain much detail and are difficult to summarise in a short comment. These are included in the data with the comment 'see reference for details'. However, it should be re-emphasised that readers should refer back to the original papers before deciding the shelf-life of any CIVAS product.

7.2 References

1. Medicines Control Agency. Guidance to the NHS on the licensing requirements of the Medicines Act 1968. London: Medicines Control Agency, 1992.

2. Farwell J. Aseptic dispensing for NHS patients. London: Department of Health, 1994.

3. The stability of drugs in syringes and bags: a collaborative study by hospital quality control staff. Pharm J 1992; 248(Suppl): HS24-HS26.

4. Adams PS, et al. Pharmaceutical aspects of home infusion therapy for cancer patients. Pharm J 1987; 238: 476-8.

5. The stability of drugs in syringes and bags: a collaborative study by hospital quality control staff. Pharm J 1992; 249(Suppl): HS20-HS21.

6. Savello DR, Shangraw RF. Stability of sodium ampicillin solutions in the frozen and liquid states. Am J Hosp Pharm 1971; 28: 754-9.

7. Bundgaard H. Polymerization of penicillins: kinetics and mechanism of polymerization of ampicillin in aqueous solution. Acta Pharm Suec 1976; 13: 9-26.

7.3 Summary of Stability Data

Product	Container	Shelf-life	Reference
Acetazolamide 375mg/L in NaCl 0.9% or in glucose 5%	Bag	7% loss in 5 days at 25°C and 5% loss in 44 days at 5°C	Am J Hosp Pharm 1987; 44: 358-60
Aciclovir 250mg/10mL in NaCl 0.9%	Syringe	Crystallises after 2 days in fridge, t90% 4 days at room temperature	Pharm J 1992; 248(Suppl): HS20-1
Aciclovir 500mg/100mL in NaCl 0.9%	Bag	28 days at room temperature or 4°C	Pharm J 1992; 248(Suppl): HS20-1
Aciclovir 5g/L in NaCl 0.9% or in glucose 5%	Bag	No loss in 37 days at 25°C and 5°C but could precipitate at 5°C	J Clin Pharm Ther 1989; 14: 451-6
Aciclovir in glucose 5% and in NaCl 0.9%	Pump (PVC)	Stable for 37 days at room temperature and 4°C	Trissel
Adrenaline 1:200000 in fentanyl/bupivacaine	Bag	Adrenaline 2.3% loss in 56 days at 4°C, 37.3% loss at 35°C	Br J Anaesth 1992; 68: 414-7
Alfentanil 25mg/50mL in glucose 5%	Syringe	No significant loss after 16 weeks at room temperature and 8°C	Pharm Pract 1995; 5: 303-4
Alfentanil 0.05% and midazolam 0.02% in NaCl 0.9%	Syringe	Alfentanil <5% degradation after 6 weeks at 6°C and room temperature. Midazolam <10% degradation after 3 weeks at room temperature and 4 weeks at 6°C.	Pharm Pract 1997; 7: 305-8
Alfentanil and propofol	Syringe pump	Compatible for 6 hours	Int J Pharmaceutics 1996; 127: 255-9
Amikacin 250 and 500mg/20mL in glucose 10%	Vial	No significant degradation after 30 days	Am J Hosp Pharm 1994; 51: 518-9
Amikacin 500mg in glucose 5% and in NaCl 0.9%	Bag	Stable for 48 hours at room temperature and 4°C	Am J Hosp Pharm 1991; 48: 2166-71
Amikacin <500mg/100mL in glucose 5% and in NaCl 0.9%	Pump (PVC)	Stable for 24 hours at room temperature, 60 days at 4°C	Trissel
Amikacin and ciprofloxacin 500/200mg/100mL in NaCl 0.9%	Bag	Both stable for 24 hours at room temperature and 4°C	Am J Hosp Pharm 1991; 48: 2166-71
Amikacin and ciprofloxacin 500/200mg/100mL in glucose 5%	Bag	Ciprofloxacin stable for 48 hours but amikacin only stable for 8 hours at 4°C	Am J Hosp Pharm 1991; 48: 2166-71
Amikacin and ciprofloxacin 500/200mg/100mL in glucose 5%	Bag	Both stable for 48 hours at room temperature	Am J Hosp Pharm 1991; 48: 2166-71
Amiloride hydrochloride 0.001M in NaCl 0.9%	Syringe	Stable for 30 days at 4°C	Pharm J 1992; 248(Suppl): HS40-1
Aminophylline 200mg in glucose 5% and in NaCl 0.9%	Bag	Stable for 48 hours at room temperature and 4°C	Am J Hosp Pharm 1991; 48: 2166-71
Aminophylline 250mg/50mL in NaCl 0.9%	Syringe	No significant loss after 6 weeks at 4°C and room temperature	Pharm J 1992; 248(Suppl): HS24-6
Aminophylline and ranitidine in NaCl 0.9%	Bag (PVC)	Stable for 48 hours	Am J Hosp Pharm 1994; 51: 1802-7
Aminophylline and ceftriaxone in NaCl 0.9%	Bag	Stable for only 2 hours at a concentration of 4 and 20mg/mL	Am J Hosp Pharm 1994; 51: 92-4
Aminophylline and ceftriaxone in glucose 5%	Bag	Stable for <24 hours at 1, 4, 20, and 40mg/mL	Am J Hosp Pharm 1994; 51: 92-4
Aminophylline and ciprofloxacin 200mg/100mL	Bag	Precipitates in 4 hours, in NaCl and in glucose 5%, at room temperature and 4°C	Am J Hosp Pharm 1991; 48: 2166-71
Amiodarone in NaCl 0.9%	Bag	Precipitates in 24 hours	Am J Hosp Pharm 1985; 42: 2679-82
Amiodarone in glucose 5%	Bag	10% loss in 3 hours due to adsorption	Am J Hosp Pharm 1985; 42: 2679-82
Amoxycillin 10mg/mL in NaCl 0.9%	Glass	<3% loss in 24 hours at 0°C	Aust J Hosp Pharm 1989; 19: 194-7
Amoxycillin 10, 20, 50mg/mL in NaCl 0.9%	Glass	3% and 7% loss in 6 hours and 12% in 4 hours at 25°C	J Clin Hosp Pharm 1982; 7: 245-50
Amoxycillin 10, 20, 50mg/mL in glucose 5%	Glass	14% and 18% loss in 3 hours and 14% in 1.5 hours at 25°C	J Clin Hosp Pharm 1982; 7: 245-50
Amoxycillin 1mg/mL in NaCl 0.9%	Glass	10% loss in 24 hours at room temperature	Farmaco (Prat) 1982; 37: 185-8
Amoxycillin 1mg/mL in glucose 5%	Glass	9% loss in 4 hours and 34% in 24 hours at room temperature	Farmaco (Prat) 1982; 37: 185-8
Amoxycillin and clavulanic acid in glucose 5%	Bag	1.2 hours in fridge	Pharm J 1987; 238: 116
Amoxycillin and clavulanic acid in compound sodium lactate	Bag	3 hours at room temperature	Pharm J 1987; 238: 116
Amoxycillin and clavulanic acid M/6 compound sodium lactate	Bag	4 hours at room temperature	Pharm J 1987; 238: 116
Amoxycillin and clavulanic acid in NaCl 0.9% 120mL	Bag	12.5 hours in fridge, 5 hours at room temperature	Pharm J 1987; 238: 116
Amoxycillin and clavulanic acid in NaCl with KCl	Bag	3 hours at room temperature	Pharm J 1987; 238: 116
Amoxycillin and clavulanic acid in Ringer's solution	Bag	3 hours at room temperature	Pharm J 1987; 238: 116
Amoxycillin and clavulanic acid in water 120mL	Bag	15 hours in fridge, 4 hours at room temperature	Pharm J 1987; 238: 116
Amphotericin B 1mg/mL in water	Bottle	No significant loss after 30 days at room temperature and in the refrigerator	Eur J Hosp Pharm 1997; 3: 59-60
Amphotericin B 5mg/mL in water	Vial	24 hours at room temperature, 7 days in fridge	ABPI. Data sheet 1996-7

Amphotericin B 0.2 and 0.5mg/mL in glucose 5%	Bag	Stable for 120 hours at 4°C and 25°C	Am J Hosp Pharm 1994; 51: 394-6
Amphotericin B 0.52-0.81mg/mL in glucose 5%	Bag	No significant loss after 24 hours at 25°C	Am J Hosp Pharm 1991; 48: 1691
Amphotericin B 0.05 and 0.5mg/mL in glucose 5%	Bag (PVC)	Stable for 24 hours at room temperature	Am J Health-Syst Pharm 1997; 54: 683-6
Amphotericin 0.1 and 0.25mg/mL in glucose 5%	Bag	No significant loss at 4°C after 35 days	Am J Hosp Pharm 1991; 48: 2635-7
Amphotericin B 0.5, 1 and 2mg/mL in lipid 20%	Glass	Challenges *ibid* 2724, artefact after redispersion?	Am J Health-Syst Pharm 1996; 53: 2701
Amphotericin B 0.5, 1 and 2mg/mL in lipid 20%	Glass	Yellow precipitate at 4 hours, redispersed, stable for 7 days at room temperature	Am J Health-Syst Pharm 1996; 53: 2724-7
Amphotericin B 1mg/mL in glucose 5%	Bag	Turbid but chemically stable for 120 hours at 4°C and 25°C	Am J Hosp Pharm 1994; 51: 394-6
Amphotericin B 45mg/500mL in lipid 20%	Bag	Stable for 1 hour, after 6 hours only 56% remains	Ann Pharmacother 1996; 30: 298
Amphotericin B 0.05 and 0.5mg/mL in lipid	Bag (PVC)	Stable for 24 hours at room temperature although separation occurred	Am J Health-Syst Pharm 1997; 54: 683-6
Amphotericin B 5mg/50mL in glucose 10%	Bag	Stable for 24 hours at 25°C, no significant loss	Am J Hosp Pharm 1991; 48: 2430-3
Amphotericin B 5mg/50mL in glucose 5%	Bag	Stable for 24 hours at 25°C, no significant loss	Am J Hosp Pharm 1991; 48: 2430-3
Amphotericin B 5mg/50mL in glucose 20%	Bag	Stable for 24 hours at 25°C, no significant loss	Am J Hosp Pharm 1991; 48: 2430-3
Amphotericin B 5mg/50mL in glucose 5%	Bag	Stable for 24 hours at 25°C, no significant loss	Am J Hosp Pharm 1991; 48: 2430-3
Amphotericin B 45mg/500mL in lipid	Bottle	56% loss in 6 hours	Ann Pharmacother 1996; 30: 298
Amphotericin B 60, 80 and 100mg/50mL in glucose 5%	Bag	>36 hours at 6°C and 25°C	Am J Hosp Pharm1991; 48: 283-5
Ampicillin	Bag	Concentration dependent	Trissel
Ampicillin	Syringe	Concentration dependent	Trissel
Ampicillin 0.5% in NaCl 0.9%	Bag	4 days in fridge, use within 6 hours at room temperature	Pharm J 1992; 248(Suppl): HS20-1
Ampicillin 0.5, 1% in NaCl 0.9%	Bag	24 and 48 hours for 10% loss at 5°C	Int J Pharmaceutics 1993; 97: 219-20
Ampicillin 0.5, 1% in NaCl 0.9%	Bag	t90% 12.2 and 6.8 days at 5°C	Int J Pharmaceutics 1993; 97: 219-20
Ampicillin 1% in NaCl 0.9%	Bag	2 days in fridge, use within 6 hours at room temperature	Pharm J 1992; 248(Suppl): HS20-1
Ampicillin 20mg/mL in NaCl 0.9%	Pump reservoir	Loss of 4% in 8 hours at 25°C, and 7% in 3 days at 5°C	Am J Health-Syst Pharm 1996; 53: 2740-3
Ampicillin 250mg/1.8mL in water (0.2mL/syringe)	Syringe	Not recommended, 36% loss in 48 hours in fridge	Hosp Pharm Pract 1992; 2: 285-9
Ampicillin 2.5% in water	Syringe	3 days in fridge, 24 hours at room temperature	Pharm J 1992; 248(Suppl): HS20-1
Ampicillin 5% in water	Syringe	Use within 6 hours of preparation	Pharm J 1992; 248(Suppl): HS20-1
Ampicillin 60mg/mL in NaCl 0.9%	Pump reservoir	24 hours at 5°C, 6 hours at 30°C	Am J Hosp Pharm 1995; 52: 70-4
Ampicillin 60mg/mL in water	Pump reservoir	24 hours at 5°C, 6 hours at 30°C	Am J Hosp Pharm 1995; 52: 70-4
Ampicillin in glucose 5% and in NaCl 0.9%	Pump (PVC)	In glucose, 4 hours at room temperature and 4°C. In NaCl, 24 hours at room temperature and 5 days at 4°C.	Trissel
Ampicillin 20mg/sulbactam 10mg/mL in NaCl 0.9%	Bag	10% loss in ampicillin 60 hours at 5°C, 24 hours at 24°C; sulbactam stable.	Am J Hosp Pharm 1994; 51: 901-4
Ampicillin/aztreonam/sulbactam/ in NaCl 0.9%	Bag	10% loss in ampicillin 84 hours at 5°C, 30 hours at 24°C; rest stable.	Am J Hosp Pharm 1994; 51: 901-4
Ampicillin/sulbactam in glucose 5% and in NaCl 0.9%	Pump (PVC)	In glucose, 2 hours at room temperature, 4 hours at 4°C. In NaCl, 8 hours at room temperature, 48 hours at 4°C.	Trissel
Artesunate 30mg, sodium bicarbonate 1% 0.5mL and 50mL NaCl	Bag	t90% 9°C 130 hours, 23°C 10.6 hours, 36.5°C 1.6 hours	J Pharm Pharmacol 1996; 48: 22-6
Artesunate 60mg, sodium bicarbonate 1% 1mL and 10mL NaCl	Syringe	t90% 9°C 130 hours, 23°C 10.6 hours, 36.5°C 1.6 hours	J Pharm Pharmacol 1996; 48: 22-6
Atracurium 25mg/2.5mL	Syringe	No significant loss after 21 days at 4°C	Pharm J 1992; 248(Suppl): HS24-6
Atropine 0.6mg/mL	Syringe	No significant loss after 21 days at 4°C	Pharm J 1992; 248(Suppl): HS24-6
Azathioprine 100mg/10mL in water	Syringe	No loss at room temperature after 16 days but precipitates after 4 days at 4°C	Am J Hosp Pharm 1981; 38: 871-5
Azathioprine 2g/L in NaCl 0.9%	Bag	Stable for 16 days at 23°C and 4°C	Am J Hosp Pharm 1981; 38: 871-5
Azathioprine 2g/L in glucose 5%	Bag	Stable for 8 days at 23°C and 4°C precipitate in 16 days	Am J Hosp Pharm 1981; 38: 871-5
Azlocillin 5g in 100mL in NaCl 0.9%	Bag	6 days in a fridge use within 3 days at room temperature	Pharm J 1992; 248(Suppl): HS40-1
Aztreonam 10mg/mL in NaCl 0.9%	Bag	No significant degradation after 96 hours at 24°C and 5°C	Am J Hosp Pharm 1994; 51: 901-4
Aztreonam 60mg/mL in water	Pump	6% loss in 70 days at 4°C, 0% at -20°C, 8% in 72 hours at 37°C	Pharm World Sci 1996; 18: 74-77
Aztreonam 40mg and vancomycin 10mg/mL	Bag (PVC)	Incompatible in glucose 5% and in NaCl 0.9%	Am J Hosp Pharm 1995; 52: 2560-4
Aztreonam 4mg and vancomycin 1mg/mL in NaCl 0.9%	Bag (PVC)	31 days at 4°C and 23°C and 7 days at 32°C	Am J Hosp Pharm 1995; 52: 2560-4

Aztreonam 4mg and vancomycin 1mg/mL in glucose 5%	Bag (PVC)	31 days at 4°C,14 days at 23°C and 7 days at 32°C	Am J Hosp Pharm 1995; 52: 2560-4
Aztreonam 60mg/mL	Pump reservoir	Stable for >8 days at 5°C and 24 hours at room temperature, 6 months at -20°C	Pharm World Sci 1996; 18: 74-77
Aztreonam in glucose 5% or in NaCl 0.9%	Pump (PVC)	48 hours at room temperature, 7 days in fridge	Trissel
Aztreonam and others	Y-site	See reference for details	Am J Health-Syst Pharm 1995; 52: 1086-90
Aztreonam/ampicillin/sulbactam in NaCl 0.9%	Bag	10% loss in ampicillin 84 hours at 5°C, 30 hours at 24°C, rest stable	Am J Hosp Pharm 1994; 51: 901-4
Baclofen 10mg,morphine 50mg/50mL in NaCl 0.9%	Pump	No significant degradation after 30 days at 37°C	Int J Pharmaceutics 1995; 118: 181-9
Baclofen 50µg/mL in NaCl 0.9%	Syringe	2 months at room temperature and 4°C	Pharm J 1992; 248(Suppl): HS40-1
Baclofen and morphine	Pump	Stable for >30 days at 37°C	Aust J Hosp Pharm 1992; 22: 258
Benzylpenicillin 1.2g/100mL in NaCl 0.9%	Bag	2 days in fridge, use within 24 hours at room temperature	Pharm J 1992; 248(Suppl): HS20-1
Benzylpenicillin 600mg/3.6mL water	Syringe	Stable for 8 days in fridge	Hosp Pharm Pract 1991; 1: 243-252
Bleomycin 0.3u/mL in NaCl 0.9%	Bag	<1% loss in 24 hours at 20°C	Am J Hosp Pharm 1990; 47: 2528-9
Bleomycin 0.3u/mL in NaCl 0.9%	Vial	<1% loss in 24 hours at 20°C	Am J Hosp Pharm 1990; 47: 2528-9
Bleomycin 0.3u/mL in glucose 5%	Bag	10% loss in 8 hours, 12% in 24 hours at 20°C	Am J Hosp Pharm 1990; 47: 2528-9
Bleomycin 0.3u/mL in glucose 5%	Vial	10% loss in 9 hours, 14% in 25 hours	Am J Hosp Pharm 1990; 47: 2528-9
Bleomycin 300 and 3000u/L in glucose 5%	Bag	10% loss in 8 hours and 11-16.5% in 24 hours at 23°C	Am J Hosp Pharm 1990; 47: 2528-9
Bleomycin 3u/mL in NaCl 0.9%	Bag	5% loss in 24 hours at 20°C	Am J Hosp Pharm 1990; 47: 2528-9
Bleomycin 3u/mL in NaCl 0.9%	Vial	2% loss in 24 hours at 20°C	Am J Hosp Pharm 1990; 47: 2528-9
Bleomycin 3u/mL in glucose 5%	Bag	9% loss in 7 hours,11% in 24 hours at 20°C	Am J Hosp Pharm 1990; 47: 2528-9
Bleomycin 3u/mL in glucose 5%	Vial	8% loss in 9 hours 16% in 25 hours	Am J Hosp Pharm 1990; 47: 2528-9
Bretylium 10g/L in glucose 5% or in NaCl 0.9%	Bag	Stable for 48 hours at room temperature and 7 days at 4°C	Am J Hosp Pharm 1981; 38: 1919-22
Bretylium 1g/L in glucose 5% or in NaCl 0.9%	Bag	Stable for 30 days at 25°C	Am J Hosp Pharm 1983; 40: 1010-12
Bumetanide 0.2 and 0.02mg/mL in glucose 5%	Bag (PVC)	Stable for 72 hours at 23-25°C	Am J Health-Syst Pharm 1997; 54: 422-3
Bupivacaine 0.125% and iohexol 300mg		No loss in 24 hours at room temperature	Pharm Weekbl (Sci) 1991; 13: 254
Bupivacaine 0.15%, diamorphine 0.02mg/mL	Bag	In NaCl, 14 days at 7°C; 5% loss of diamorphine after 24 hours at 45°C	Pharm World Sci 1995; 17: 87-92
Bupivacaine 0.1% and fentanyl 4µg/mL in NaCl 0.9%	Bag	12% loss of fentanyl; 5% loss of bupivacaine in 3 days, no further loss in 56 days	Br J Anaesth 1992; 68: 414-7
Bupivacaine 0.1% and fentanyl 5µg/mL in NaCl 0.9%	Bag	14 days at room temperature	Hosp Pharm Pract 1992; 2: 529-31
Bupivacaine 0.1% in 100mL in NaCl 0.9%	Bag	9% loss in 3 days, no further loss in 56 days at room temperature	Br J Anaesth 1992; 68: 414-7
Bupivacaine 0.1% and fentanyl 2µg/mL in NaCl 0.9%	Syringe	12 weeks at 8°C and room temperature	Pharm Pract 1995; 5: 21-22
Bupivacaine 0.1% and fentanyl 2µg/mL in NaCl 0.9%	Bag (PVC)	12 weeks at 8°C and room temperature	Pharm Pract 1995; 5: 21-22
Bupivacaine 0.25% and iohexol 300mg		No loss in 24 hours at room temperature	Pharm Weekbl (Sci) 1991; 13: 254
Bupivacaine and morphine in NaCl 0.9%	Bag (PVC)	Stable at 625-1250mg/L and 100-500mg/L for 72 hours at room temperature	Am J Health-Syst Pharm 1997; 54: 61-4
Bupivacaine 0.3% and sufentanil 20µg/mL	Cassette	No significant loss after 10 days at 26°C	Eur Hosp Pharm 1995; 1: 12-14
Bupivacaine 1.25mg/mL in NaCl 0.9%	Syringe	Stable for at least 32 days at 3°C and 25°C	Am J Hosp Pharm 1993; 50: 2364-5
Bupivacaine and adrenaline and fentanyl	Pump	Fentanyl and bupivacaine no significant loss at 3°C after 30 days	Am J Hosp Pharm 1993; 50: 714-5
Calcitrol 0.5µg/mL in glucose 5%, NaCl 0.9% and water	Syringe	Stable for 8 hours at room temperature in light	Am J Hosp Pharm 1992; 49: 1463-6
Carbenicillin glucose 5% or in NaCl 0.9%	Pump (PVC)	24 hours at room temperature, 72 hours in fridge	Trissel
Carboplatin 0.8 and 3.2mg/mL in glucose 5%	Glass	Under diffuse light in NaCl 0.9% t90% 1-10 hours	Int J Pharmaceutics 1996; 129: 275-7
Carboplatin 100mg and fluorouracil 1g/L in glucose 5%	Bag	16% loss of carboplatin at room temperature	J Clin Pharm Ther 1994; 19: 127-33
Carboplatin 100mg and fluorouracil 1g/L in glucose 5%	Bag	2.8% loss of carboplatin at room temperature after 2 days (buffered)	J Clin Pharm Ther 1994; 19: 127-33
Carboplatin 3.2mg/mL in glucose 5%	Bag	No significant degradation after 30 days at 25°C	J Pharm Biomed Anal 1994; 12: 81-4
Carboplatin 3.2mg/mL in glucose 5%	Bottle	No significant degradation after 30 days at 25°C	J Pharm Biomed Anal 1994; 12: 81-4
Carboplatin 6 and 10mg/mL	Pump	Stable for 14 days at 37°C	J Pharm Biomed Anal 1993; 11: 723-7
Carboplatin 600mg/250mL in glucose 5%	Bag	No significant loss after 9 days at room temperature	J Clin Pharm Ther 1994; 19: 95-100
Cefapirin in glucose 5% or in NaCl 0.9%	Pump (PVC)	24 hours at room temperature, 10 days in fridge	Trissel

Cefmetazole 1g and doxycycline 100-200mg in glucose 5%	Bag (PVC)	Cefmetazole 72 hours, 5% degradation; doxycycline stable at room temperature for 96 hours; both <10% degradation after 168 hours at 4°C	J Clin Pharm Ther 1994; 19: 317-25
Cefmetazole 1g and doxycycline 100-200mg in NaCl 0.9%	Bag (PVC)	Cefmetazole <4 hours, doxycycline stable at room temperature; both <10% degradation after 168 hours at 4°C followed by 8 hours at room temperature	J Clin Pharm Ther 1994; 19: 317-25
Cefmetazole 1 and 2g/100 and 250mL in NaCl 0.9%	Bag (PVC)	Stable for 48 hours; 8% loss at room temperature and 168 hours, and at 4°C and 8 hours at room temperature	J Clin Pharm Ther 1994; 19: 317-25
Cefmetazole 1 and 2g/100 and 250mL in glucose 5%	Bag (PVC)	Stable for 24 hours; 5% loss at room temperature and 168 hours, and at 4°C and 8 hours at room temperature	J Clin Pharm Ther 1994; 19: 317-25
Cefmetazole 2g and doxycycline 100mg in glucose 5%	Bag (PVC)	Precipitate in 8 hours at 4°C,<10% loss at room temperature after 96 hours	J Clin Pharm Ther 1994; 19: 317-25
Cefmetazole 2g and doxycycline 100mg in NaCl 0.9%	Bag (PVC)	Precipitate in 48 hours at 4°C, 10% loss at room temperature after 8 hours	J Clin Pharm Ther 1994; 19: 317-25
Cefmetazole 5mg and famotidine 0.2mg/mL in glucose 5%	IV set	168 hours at 4°C and 120 hours at 25°C	Am J Hosp Pharm 1996; 53: 432-3
Cefonicid in glucose 5% or in NaCl 0.9%	Pump (PVC)	24 hours at room temperature, 72 hours in fridge	Trissel
Cefoperazone 300mg/mL in water	Syringe	24 hours at room temperature 5 days at 2-8°C	Trissel
Cefoperazone 5mg, cimetidine 2mg/mL in glucose 5%	Bag	95.5% cefoperazone and 97% cimetidine remain after 48 hours at 4°C and 25°C	Am J Hosp Pharm 1991; 48: 111-3
Cefoperazone in glucose 5% or in NaCl 0.9%	Pump (PVC)	24 hours at room temperature, 5 days in fridge	Trissel
Cefotaxime 100mg and vancomycin 25 and 50mg/mL	Y-site	Incompatible	Am J Hosp Pharm 1993; 50: 2057-8
Cefotaxime 100mg, vancomycin 5-50mg/mL	Glass	Immediate precipitate 25 and 50mg/mL	Am J Hosp Pharm 1993; 50: 2054-7
Cefotaxime 1g, metronidazole 500mg/100mL	Bag	96 hours at 4°C	Am J Health-Syst Pharm 1995; 52: 1561-3
Cefotaxime 1g/3.4mL in water (0.18mL syringe)	Syringe	7 days in fridge but increased coloration	Hosp Pharm Pract 1992; 2: 285-9
Cefotaxime in glucose 5% or in NaCl 0.9%	Pump (PVC)	24 hours at room temperature, 5 days in fridge	Trissel
Cefotetan 2mg/mL in glucose 5%	Bag	3% loss in 14 days at 4°C and 20°C	Am J Hosp Pharm 1983; 40: 1024-5
Cefotetan 95-500mg/mL in water	Syringe	24 hours at room temperature 96 hours at 2-8°C	Trissel
Cefoxitin 20mg/mL in NaCl 0.9%	Bag	No loss in 24 hours,12% in 48 hours at room temperature, 3% in 13 days at 5°C	Am J Hosp Pharm 1981; 38: 875-9
Cefoxitin 20mg/mL in glucose 5%	Bag	No loss in 24 hours, 11% in 48 hours at room temperature, 3% in 13 days at 5°C	Am J Hosp Pharm 1981; 38: 875-9
Cefoxitin in glucose 5% or in NaCl 0.9%	Pump (PVC)	48 hours at room temperature, 7 days in fridge	Trissel
Ceftazidime 100 and 200mg/mL in water	Syringe	Stable for >96 hours at 4°C and >8 hours at room temperature	Am J Hosp Pharm 1992; 49: 2765-8
Ceftazidime 100mg/L	Bag	Stable for 7 days at 4°C then 16 hours at 25°C and 8 hours at 37°C	Am J Health-Syst Pharm 1996; 53: 2731-4
Ceftazidime 100mg/mL in water	Syringe	No significant degradation in 8 hours at room temperature or 96 hours at 4°C	Am J Hosp Pharm 1992; 49: 2765-8
Ceftazidime 100mg/mL in water	Vial	No significant degradation in 96 hours at 4°C or 8 hours at room temperature	Am J Hosp Pharm 1992; 49: 2765-8
Ceftazidime 1g and metronidazole 500mg/100mL	Bag (PVC)	No significant loss of either at 8°C after 72 hours	Am J Hosp Pharm 1995; 52: 2568-70
Ceftazidime 1g/250mL in NaCl 0.9%	Bag (PVC)	No significant degradation after 24 hours at room temperature and 7 days at 4°C	Pharmazie 1994; 49: 425-7
Ceftazidime 1g/250mL in glucose 5%	Bag (PVC)	No significant degradation after 24 hours at room temperature and 7 days at 4°C	Pharmazie 1994; 49: 425-7
Ceftazidime 200mg/mL in water	Syringe	5% degradation in 96 hours at 4°C or in 8 hours at room temperature	Am J Hosp Pharm 1992; 49: 2765-8
Ceftazidime 200mg/mL in water	Vial	4% degradation in 96 hours at 4°C or in 8 hours at room temperature	Am J Hosp Pharm 1992; 49: 2765-8
Ceftazidime 20mg/mL in NaCl 0.9%	Pump reservoir	4% loss after 18 hours at 25°C and 5% after 7 days at 5°C	Am J Health-Syst Pharm 1996; 53: 2740-3
Ceftazidime 20mg/mL in glucose 5%	Pump reservoir	9% loss after 18 hours at 25°C and 5% after 7 days at 5°C	Am J Health-Syst Pharm 1996; 53: 2740-3
Ceftazidime 30mg/mL with arginine	Pump reservoir	3% loss after 10 days at 3°C	Am J Hosp Pharm 1992; 49: 2761-4
Ceftazidime 3-6g/50mL in NaCl 0.9%	Infusor	Stable for 144 hours at 4°C, t90% at 27°C 24 hours	Am J Health-Syst Pharm 1995; 52: 1912-4
Ceftazidime 500mg/4.5mL in water (0.4mL syringe)	Syringe	7 days in fridge but increased coloration	Hosp Pract 1992; 2: 285-9
Ceftazidime 60mg/mL with arginine	Pump reservoir	3% loss after 10 days at 3°C	Am J Hosp Pharm 1992; 49: 2761-4
Ceftazidime in glucose 5% or in NaCl 0.9%	Pump (PVC)	24 hours at room temperature,7 days in fridge	Trissel
Ceftazidime and aminophylline in NaCl 0.9%	Bag	Incompatible over a 24 hours period	Ann Pharmacother 1993; 26: 1221-6
Ceftazidime and arginine 100mg/mL	Syringe	No significant loss in 10 days at 4°C then 7% loss at room temperature in 24 hours	Am J Hosp Pharm 1992; 49: 2954-6

Ceftazidime and teicoplanin 100 and 25mg/L	Bag	Unstable at 25°C in paediatric dialysis solution	Am J Health-Syst Pharm 1996; 53: 2731-4
Ceftizoxime 10mg/mL in metronidazole 0.5%	Bag (PVC)	Stable for 14 days at 4°C followed by 3 days at 25°C	Am J Health-Syst Pharm 1996; 53: 1046-8
Ceftizoxime 10mg/mL in metronidazole 0.5%	Bag (PVC)	Stable for 14 days at 4°C and 3 days at room temperature	Am J Health-Syst Pharm 1996; 53: 1046-7
Ceftizoxime 1g and metronidazole 500mg/100mL	Bag (PVC)	No significant loss of either at 8°C after 72 hours	Am J Hosp Pharm 1995; 52: 2568-70
Ceftizoxime 1g/50mL in NaCl 0.9% or in glucose 5%	Bag	10% loss after 30 days at 4°C, 7 days at room temperature	Can J Hosp Pharm 1993; 46: 13-16
Ceftizoxime 20 and 40g/L in glucose 5% and in NaCl 0.9%	Bag	Stable for 48 hours at room temperature and 7 days at 5°C	Drug Intell Clin Pharm 1989; 23: 615-8
Ceftizoxime 2g/30mL in water	Syringe	9% loss in 24 hours at room temperature and in 5 days at 5°C	Drug Intell Clin Pharm 1989; 23: 615-8
Ceftizoxime in glucose 5% or in NaCl 0.9%	Pump (PVC)	24 hours at room temperature,48 hours in fridge	Trissel
Ceftizoxime, ceftriaxone, ceftazidime, metronidazole		See reference for details	Am J Health-Syst Pharm 1995; 52: 2568-70
Ceftriaxone 100mg/mL	Syringe	<10% loss in 13 days in fridge	Eur J Hosp Pharm 1996; 2: 47-8
Ceftriaxone 100mg/mL in water	Syringe	91% remains after 40 days at 4°C and 5 days at 20°C	Am J Health-Syst Pharm 1996; 53: 2320-3
Ceftriaxone 10, 40mg/mL in NaCl 0.9%	Syringe	5% loss after 48 hours at 4°C or room temperature after 10 days at -15°C	Am J Hosp Pharm 1993; 50: 2092-4
Ceftriaxone 10, 40mg/mL in glucose 5%	Syringe	No loss after 48 hours at 4°C or room temperature after 10 days at -15°C	Am J Hosp Pharm 1993; 50: 2092-4
Ceftriaxone 1g and metronidazole 500mg/100mL	Bag (PVC)	No significant loss of either at 8°C after 72 hours	Am J Hosp Pharm 1995; 52: 2568-70
Ceftriaxone 20mg/mL in NaCl 0.9%	Pump reservoir	2% loss after 72 hours at 25°C and 10 days at 5°C	Am J Health-Syst Pharm 1996; 53: 2740-3
Ceftriaxone 20mg/mL in glucose 5%	Pump reservoir	2% loss after 72 hours at 25°C and 5% after 10 days at 5°C	Am J Health-Syst Pharm 1996; 53: 2740-3
Ceftriaxone 250mg/mL in glucose 5%	Syringe	Stable for 8 weeks at -15°C then 1 day at 20°C	Am J Hosp Pharm 1994; 51: 2159-61
Ceftriaxone 40g/L in NaCl 0.9%	Bag	5% loss in 3 days at 23°C, 9% loss in 30 days at 4°C	Can J Hosp Pharm 1987; 40: 161-6
Ceftriaxone 40g/L in glucose 5%	Bag	12% loss in 3 days at 23°C, 10% loss in 14 days at 4°C	Can J Hosp Pharm 1987; 40: 161-6
Ceftriaxone in glucose 5% or in NaCl 0.9%	Pump (PVC)	72 hours at room temperature, 10 days in fridge	Trissel
Ceftriaxone 250-450mg/mL in lignocaine 1%	Syringe	8% loss at 4°C after 35 days and after 2 days at room temperature	Am J Health-Syst Pharm 1996; 53: 2323-5
Ceftriaxone and aminophylline in NaCl 0.9%	Bag	Stable for only 2 hours at concentration of 20 and 4mg/mL	Am J Hosp Pharm 1994; 51: 92-4
Ceftriaxone and aminophylline in glucose 5%	Bag	Stable for <24 hours at 20, 40 and 1, 4mg/mL	Am J Hosp Pharm 1994; 51: 92-4
Cefuroxime 1.5g and metronidazole 0.5%, 100mL	Bag	1 month stability given, pH dependent	Pharm Pract 1995; 5: 100-106
Cefuroxime 1.5g/250mL in NaCl 0.9%	Bag (PVC)	No significant degradation after 24 hours at room temperature and 7 days at 4°C	Pharmazie 1994; 49: 425-7
Cefuroxime 1.5g/250mL in glucose 5%	Bag (PVC)	No significant degradation after 24 hours at room temperature and 7 days at 4°C	Pharmazie 1994; 49: 425-7
Cefuroxime 22.5mg/mL	Pump reservoir	No significant loss after 7 days at 3°C	Am J Hosp Pharm 1992; 49: 2761-4
Cefuroxime 250mg/1.8mL in water (0.2mL syringe)	Syringe	7 days in fridge but increased coloration	Hosp Pharm Pract 1992; 2: 285-9
Cefuroxime 45mg/mL	Pump reservoir	No significant loss after 7 days at 3°C	Am J Hosp Pharm 1992; 49: 2761-4
Cefuroxime 750mg and 1.5g in 50mL of NaCl 0.9%	Bag	20 days at 4°C, use within 24 hours at room temperature	Pharm J 1992; 248(Suppl): HS40-1
Cefuroxime 750mg and 1.5g in 50mL of glucose 5%	Bag	20 days at 4°C, use within 24 hours at room temperature	Pharm J 1992; 248(Suppl): HS40-1
Cefuroxime 750mg and metronidazole 0.5%, 100mL	Bag	1 month stability given, pH dependent	Pharm Pract 1995; 5: 100-106
Cefuroxime 750mg/metronidazole 500mg	Bag	7 days at 4°C	J Clin Pharm Ther 1990; 15: 187-96
Cefuroxime/aminophylline in various fluids	Vial	Only 4 hours data at room temperature, stable for this time	Am J Hosp Pharm 1994; 51: 809-11
Cephaloridine 1g/250mL in NaCl 0.9%	Bag (PVC)	No significant degradation after 24 hours at room temperature and 7 days at 4°C	Pharmazie 1994; 49: 425-7
Cephaloridine 1g/250mL in glucose 5%	Bag (PVC)	No significant degradation after 24 hours at room temperature and 7 days at 4°C	Pharmazie 1994; 49: 425-7
Cephalothin in glucose 5% or in NaCl 0.9%	Pump (PVC)	24 hours at room temperature, 96 hours in fridge	Trissel
Cephamandole	Syringe	Not recommended as carbon dioxide in formulation blows out barrel	Am J Hosp Pharm 1979; 36: 1025
Cephamandole 20mg/mL in NaCl 0.9%	Bag	3% loss in 1 day and 6% in 5 days at 24°C, 1 and 6% in 4 days and 44 days at4°C	Am J Hosp Pharm 1981; 38: 875-9
Cephamandole 20mg/mL in NaCl 0.9%	Bag	3-4% loss in 72 hours at 25°C, 0-3% loss in 10 days at 5°C	Am J Hosp Pharm 1982; 39: 622-7
Cephamandole 20mg/mL in glucose 5%	Bag	4% loss in 1 day and 10% in 5 days at 24°C, 2 and 5% in 4 days and 44 days at 4°C	Am J Hosp Pharm 1981; 38: 875-9
Cephamandole 2mg/mL in NaCl 0.9%	Bag	1% loss in 48 hours; 13% in 72 hours at 25°C, no loss in 10 days 5°C	Am J Hosp Pharm 1982; 39: 622-7
Cephazolin 1g and famotidine 20mg/100mL in glucose 5%	Burette	5% loss of cephazolin 10 hours, 5% loss of famotidine in 24 hours at 4°C, 1 hour at room temperature	Am J Hosp Pharm 1994; 51: 2205-9

Cephazolin 20mg/mL in NaCl 0.9%	Pump reservoir	3% loss after 24 hours at 25°C and 7 days at 5°C	Am J Health-Syst Pharm 1996; 53: 2740-3
Cephazolin 20mg/mL in glucose 5%	Pump reservoir	No significant loss after 24 hours at 25°C and 2% after 7 days at 5°C	Am J Health-Syst Pharm 1996; 53: 2740-3
Cephradine 0.5g/100mL in NaCl 0.9%	Bag	7 days in fridge, use within 48 hours at room temperature	Pharm J 1992; 248(Suppl): HS20-1
Cephradine in glucose 5% or in NaCl 0.9%	Pump (PVC)	10 hours at room temperature, 48 hours in fridge	Trissel
Chloramphenicol in glucose 5%	Pump (PVC)	30 days at room temperature	Trissel
Cidofovir 0.21 and 8.12mg/mL in NaCl 0.9%	Bag (PVC)	Stable for 24 hours in fridge and 30°C	Am J Health-Syst Pharm 1996; 53: 1939-43
Cidofovir 0.21 and 8.12mg/mL in glucose 5%	Bag (PVC)	Stable for 24 hours in fridge and 30°C	Am J Health-Syst Pharm 1996; 53: 1939-43
Cimetidine 15mg/mL in water	Vial	Stable for 14 days at 22°C and 42 days at 4°C	Am J Hosp Pharm1993; 50: 2559-61
Cimetidine 600µg/mL in NaCl 0.9%		Stable for 48 hours at 22-26°C	Am J Hosp Pharm 1995; 52: 2024-5
Ciprofloxacin 0.8mg/mL in 250mL of NaCl 0.9%	Bag	No significant loss at room temperature in light after 6 hours	Int J Pharmaceutics 1993; 89: 125-131
Ciprofloxacin 0.8mg/mL in 250mL of glucose 5%	Bag	No significant loss at room temperature in light after 6 hours	Int J Pharmaceutics 1993; 89: 125-131
Ciprofloxacin in glucose 5% or in NaCl 0.9%	Pump (PVC)	14 days at room temperature, 14 days in fridge	Trissel
Ciprofloxacin 0.4% in NaCl 0.9%	Bag	No significant loss after 3 months at 5°C and room temperature	J Clin Pharm Ther 1994; 19: 261-2
Ciprofloxacin 0.4% in glucose 5%	Bag	No significant loss after 3 months at 5°C and room temperature	J Clin Pharm Ther 1994; 19: 261-2
Ciprofloxacin 200mg in 100mL in NaCl 0.9%	Bag	>2 days at 25°C	Am J Hosp Pharm 1991; 48: 2166-71
Ciprofloxacin 200mg in 100mL in glucose 5%	Bag	>2 days at 25°C	Am J Hosp Pharm 1991; 48: 2166-71
Ciprofloxacin 200mg/100mL in 0.5% metronidazole	Bag	Both stable for 48 hours at room temperature and 4°C	Am J Hosp Pharm 1991; 48: 2166-71
Ciprofloxacin 200mg/100mL in NaCl 0.9%	Bag	No significant loss in 48 hours under room conditions	Am J Hosp Pharm 1991; 48: 2166-71
Ciprofloxacin 200mg/100mL in glucose 5%	Bag	No significant loss in 48 hours under room conditions	Am J Hosp Pharm 1991; 48: 2166-71
Ciprofloxacin 200mg/100mL in 0.5% metronidazole	Bag	>2 days at 25°C	Am J Hosp Pharm 1991; 48: 2166-71
Ciprofloxacin 2mg/mL and 12 other drugs	Y-site	Compatible	Ann Pharmacother 1993; 27: 704-7
Ciprofloxacin 2mg/mL and frusemide 5mg/mL	Y-site	Incompatible	Ann Pharmacother 1993; 27: 704-7
Ciprofloxacin 2mg/mL and heparin 2u/mL	Y-site	Incompatible	Ann Pharmacother 1993; 27: 704-7
Ciprofloxacin 2mg/mL and teicoplanin 60mg/mL	Y-site	Incompatible	Ann Pharmacother 1993; 27: 704-7
Ciprofloxacin and amikacin 200mg/500mg/in 100mL of NaCl 0.9%	Bag	Both stable for 48 hours at room temperature and 4°C	Am J Hosp Pharm 1991; 48: 2166-71
Ciprofloxacin and amikacin 200mg/500mg/in 100mL of glucose 5%	Bag	Ciprofloxacin no loss in 48 hours, amikacin 12% loss in 24 hours at 4°C	Am J Hosp Pharm 1991; 48: 2166-71
Ciprofloxacin and amikacin 200mg/500mg/in 100mL of glucose 5%	Bag	Both stable for 48 hours at room temperature	Am J Hosp Pharm 1991; 48: 2166-71
Ciprofloxacin and aminophylline 200mg/in 100mL of NaCl 0.9%	Bag	Precipitate after 4 hours	Am J Hosp Pharm 1991; 48: 2166-71
Ciprofloxacin and aminophylline 200mg/in 100mL of glucose 5%	Bag	Precipitate after 4 hours	Am J Hosp Pharm 1991; 48: 2166-71
Ciprofloxacin and clindamycin 200mg/900mg/in 100mL of glucose 5%	Bag	In 100mL immediate precipitate	Am J Hosp Pharm 1991; 48: 2166-71
Ciprofloxacin and clindamycin 200mg/900mg/ in NaCl 0.9%	Bag	Immediate precipitate	Am J Hosp Pharm 1991; 48: 2166-71
Ciprofloxacin and gentamicin 200mg/120mg/in 100mL of glucose 5%	Bag	Stable for 48 hours at room temperature and 4°C	Am J Hosp Pharm 1991; 48: 2166-71
Ciprofloxacin and gentamicin 200mg/120mg/in NaCl 0.9%	Bag	In 100mL stable for 48 hours at room temperature and 4°C	Am J Hosp Pharm 1991; 48: 2166-71
Ciprofloxacin and tobramycin 200mg/120mg/in 100mL of NaCl 0.9%	Bag	Both stable for 24 hours at room temperature and 4°C	Am J Hosp Pharm 1991; 48: 2166-71
Ciprofloxacin and tobramycin 200mg /120mg/in 100mL in glucose 5%	Bag	Both stable for 24 hours at room temperature and 4°C	Am J Hosp Pharm 1991; 48: 2166-71
Cisplatin 0.2mg, ondansetron 0.48mg/mL	Reservoir	In NaCl 0.9% 168 hours at 2-8°C plus 24 hours at 30°C	Am J Health-Syst Pharm 1995; 52: 2570-3
Cisplatin 0.455mg, ondansetron 1.091mg/mL	Bag	In NaCl 0.9% in PVC, 24 hours 2-8°C and 168 hours at 30°C	Am J Health-Syst Pharm 1995; 52: 2570-3
Cisplatin 150mg/250mL in NaCl 0.9%	Bag	No significant loss after 9 days at room temperature	J Clin Pharm Ther 1994; 19: 95-100
Cisplatin 150mg/250mL in glucose 5%	Bag	No significant loss after 9 days at room temperature	J Clin Pharm Ther 1994; 19: 95-100
Clindamycin 15mg/mL in water	Vial	Stable for 91 days at 22°C and 4°C	Am J Hosp Pharm1993; 50: 2559-61
Clindamycin 20-120mg/mL in water	Syringe	Stable for 30 days at room temperature	Trissel

Clindamycin 750mg/mL in glucose 5%	Bag	30 days frozen and 14 days in fridge	Am J Hosp Pharm 1991; 48: 2184-6
Clindamycin 900mg in glucose 5% and in NaCl 0.9%	Bag	Stable for 48 hours at room temperature and 4°C	Am J Hosp Pharm 1991; 48: 2166-71
Clindamycin glucose 5% or in NaCl 0.9%	Pump (PVC)	16 days at room temperature, 32 days in fridge	Trissel
Clindamycin and ciprofloxacin 900/200mg/ in 100mL NaCl 0.9%	Bag	Immediate precipitate	Am J Hosp Pharm 1991; 48: 2166-71
Clindamycin and ciprofloxacin 900/200mg/ in 100mL glucose 5%	Bag	Immediate precipitate	Am J Hosp Pharm 1991; 48: 2166-71
Co-trimoxazole 96mg/mL	Syringe	No significant degradation in 60 hours at room temperature	Am J Hosp Pharm 1992; 49: 2782-3
Co-trimoxazole 96mg/mL; undiluted	Syringe	No significant loss in 60 hours under room conditions	Am J Hosp Pharm 1992; 49: 2782-3
Co-trimoxazole in NaCl 0.9%	Pump (PVC)	48 hours at room temperature	Trissel
Cyclophosphamide 0.3mg and ondansetron 0.05mg	Bag (PVC)	8 days at 4°C or 4 days at room temperature	Am J Hosp Pharm 1995; 52: 514-6
Cyclophosphamide 20mg/mL in water	Syringe	3% loss in 4 weeks at 4°C, 10% in 11 weeks	Br J Parenter Ther 1984; 5: 90-7
Cyclophosphamide 2mg and ondansetron 0.4mg/mL	Bag (PVC)	8 days at 4°C or 4 days at room temperature	Am J Hosp Pharm 1995; 52: 514-6
Cyclophosphamide 4g/L in NaCl 0.9%	Bag	No loss in 4 weeks at 4°C	Br J Par Ther 1984; 5: 90-7
Cyclophosphamide and ondansetron in NaCl 0.9%	Bag (PVC)	Stable for 8 days at 4°C and 4 days at room temperature	Am J Health-Syst Pharm 1995; 52: 514-6
Cyclophosphamide and ondansetron in glucose 5%	Bag (PVC)	Stable for 8 days at 4°C and 4 days at room temperature	Am J Health-Syst Pharm 1995; 52: 514-6
Cytarabine 1.25 and 25 mg/mL in NaCl 0.9%	Pump reservoir	28 days at 4-22°C and 7 days at 35°C	Am J Hosp Pharm 1992; 49: 619-23
Cytarabine 1.25 and 25 mg/mL in glucose 5%	Pump reservoir	28 days at 4-22°C and 7 days at 35°C	Am J Hosp Pharm 1992; 49: 619-23
Cytarabine 40/80mg/mL in water	Syringe	Stable for 15 days at 4 and 25°C, 7 days at 37°C	Trissel
Cytarabine 8/32g/L in glucose 5% and in NaCl 0.9%	Bag	Stable for 7 days at 4 and 25°C	Trissel
Cytarabine and ondansetron	Bag (PVC)	Stable for >48 hours at room temperature	Am J Health-Syst Pharm 1996; 53: 1297-1300
Dacarbazine and ondansetron 1-3, 0.03-0.3mg/L	Bag (PVC)	Stable for >48 hours at room temperature	Am J Health-Syst Pharm 1996; 53: 1297-1300
Daunorubicin 1.6mg/100mL in NaCl 0.9%	Bag	No significant loss in 7 days at 4°C	Pharm Weekbl (Sci) 1992; 14: 365-9
Daunorubicin 1.6mg/100mL in glucose 5%	Bag	No significant loss in 7 days at 4°C	Pharm Weekbl (Sci) 1992; 14: 365-9
Desferrioxamine mesylate <318mg/mL in water	Pump	Physically and chemically stable for 7 days	Can J Hosp Pharm 1994; 47: 9-14
Desferrioxamine mesylate >318mg/mL in water	Pump	Precipitates after 5 days	Can J Hosp Pharm 1994; 47: 9-14
Dexamethasone 0.2-0.4mg/ondansetron	Bag	Stable for 30 days at 4°C then 2 days at room temperature	Am J Health-Syst Pharm 1996; 53: 1431-5
Dexamethasone 10mg/ondansetron 5-32mg	Syringe	Stable for 30 days at 4°C then 2 days at room temperature	Am J Health-Syst Pharm 1996; 53: 1431-5
Dexamethasone 10-20mg/ondansetron 5-32mg	Bag (PVC)	Stable for 30 days at 4°C then 2 days at room temperature	Am J Health-Syst Pharm 1996; 53: 1431-5
Dexamethasone 1mg/mL in NaCl 0.9%	Vial	>97.7% remained after 28 days at room temperature and 4°C	Ann Pharmacother 1994; 28: 1018-9
Dexamethasone 20mg/ondansetron 8/32/in glucose 5%	Bag	Stable for 24 hours at room temperature	Am J Hosp Pharm 1993; 50: 1410-4
Dexamethasone 20mg/ondansetron 5-32mg	Syringe	In 20 and 30mL NaCl some combinations produced a precipitate	Am J Health-Syst Pharm 1996; 53: 1431-5
Dexamethasone 20mg/ondansetron 8, 32mg in NaCl 0.9%	Bag	Stable for 24 hours at room temperature	Am J Hosp Pharm 1993; 50: 1410-4
Dexamethasone 0.2-0.4mg/mL in NaCl 0.9%	Bag (PVC)	Stable for 30 days at 4°C then 2 days at room temperature	Am J Health-Syst Pharm 1996; 53: 1431-5
Dexamethasone and granisetron in NaCl 0.9%	Bag (PVC)	Stable for 14 days at room temperature or 4°C	Am J Health-Syst Pharm 1996; 53: 1174-6
Dexamethasone and granisetron in glucose 5%	Bag (PVC)	Stable for 14 days at room temperature or 4°C	Am J Health-Syst Pharm 1996; 53: 1174-6
Dexamethasone/ondansetron/lorazepam/in glucose 5%	Bag	Lorazepam loses >10% in 4 hours at room temperature	Am J Hosp Pharm 1993; 50: 1410-4
Dexamethasone/ondansetron/lorazepam/in NaCl 0.9%	Bag	Lorazepam loses >10% in 4 hours	Am J Hosp Pharm 1993; 50: 1410-4
Dexamethasone/diphenhydramine/lorazepam/metoclopramide	Pump	Lorazepam 15% loss in 24 hours, others stable for 15 days	Am J Hosp Pharm 1994; 51: 514-7
Diamorphine 0.02mg/mL, bupivacaine 0.15%	Bag	Stable for 14 days at 7°C	Pharm World Sci 1995; 17: 87-92
Diamorphine 1 and 10mg/mL and bupivacaine 0.5%	Syringe	At least 4 weeks at room temperature or 6°C	Pharm Pract 1996; 6: 113,114,118
Diamorphine 1 and 20mg/mL in NaCl 0.9%	Bag	15 days at 4 and 20°C	Am J Hosp Pharm 1990; 47: 377-81
Diamorphine 1 and 20mg/mL in NaCl 0.9%	Infusor	15 days at 4, 20 and 31°C	Am J Hosp Pharm 1990; 47: 377-81
Diamorphine 10mg, midazolam 10mg/15mL in water	Syringe	Stable for 14 days at room temperature	Int J Pharm Pract 1994; 3: 57-9
Diamorphine 400mg and chlorpromazine 25mg/10mL	Syringe	In water 9% degradation of diamorphine after 9 days	Pharm J 1992; 248(Suppl): HS24-6
Diamorphine 500mg, midazolam 75mg/15mL in water	Syringe	Stable for 14 days at room temperature	Int J Pharm Pract 1994; 3: 57-9
Diamorphine 50-150mg/hyoscine 0.4mg/mL	Syringe	Compatible with 7% diamorphine loss in 7 days at room temperature	Br J Pharm Pract 1986; 8: 218-20

Diamorphine 50-150/metoclopramide 5mg/mL	Syringe	Discoloration and 8% metoclopramide loss and 9% diamorphine loss in 7 days	Br J Pharm Pract 1986; 8: 218-20
Diamorphine and bupivacaine epidurals	PCA bag	No significant change in 8 days at room temperature	Palliative Med 1995; 9: 315-8
Diazepam 10mg/100mL in NaCl 0.9%	Bag	No significant loss in 24 hours	Int J Pharmaceutics 1994; 110: 197-201
Diazepam 10mg/100mL in NaCl 0.9%	Bag (PVC)	40% loss in 5 hours, 70% in 24 hours	Int J Pharmaceutics 1994; 110: 197-201
Diethanolamine fusidate 580mg/250mL in glucose 5%	Bag	10% degradation after 2 days at 37°C, 10 days at 25°C, >162 days at 4°C	Hosp Pharm Pract 1992; 1: 59-62
Diethanolamine fusidate 580mg/500mL in glucose 5%	Bag	10% degradation after 2 days at 37°C, 10 days at 25°C, >162 days at 4°C	Hosp Pharm Pract 1992; 1: 59-62
Diphenhydramine/lorazepam/metoclopramide/dexamethasone/ in NaCl	Pump	Lorazepam 15% loss in 24 hours, others stable for 15 days	Am J Hosp Pharm 1994; 51: 514-7
Dobutamine 250 and 500mg/50mL in NaCl 0.9%	Syringe	No significant degradation after 4 weeks at 4°C	Hosp Pharm Pract 1991; 5: 255-6
Dobutamine 250 and 500mg/50mL in glucose 5%	Syringe	No significant degradation after 4 weeks at 4°C	Hosp Pharm Pract 1991; 5: 255-6
Dobutamine 5mg/mL in glucose 5%	Syringe	48 hours at 4°C and room temperature	Am J Hosp Pharm 1996; 53: 186,193
Dobutamine and ranitidine in NaCl 0.9%	Bag (PVC)	Stable for 48 hours	Am J Hosp Pharm 1994; 51: 1802-7
Docetaxel 0.56 and 0.96mg/mL in glucose 5% and NaCl 0.9%	Bag (PVC)	Leached DEHP when stored for up to 8 hours at room temperature	Am J Health-Syst Pharm 1997; 54: 566-9
Dopamine 0.3 and 1mg/mL in glucose 10%/NaCl 0.18%	Bag	No loss over 48 hours	Pharm J 1991; 246: 220
Dopamine 0.3 and 1mg/mL in glucose 10%	Bag	No loss over 48 hours	Pharm J 1991; 246: 220
Dopamine 4mg/mL in glucose 5%	Syringe	48 hours at 4°C and room temperature	Am J Hosp Pharm 1996; 53: 186,193
Dopamine and ranitidine in NaCl 0.9%	Bag (PVC)	Stable for 48 hours	Am J Hosp Pharm 1994; 51: 1802-7
Doxorubicin 1.25 and 0.5 mg/mL in NaCl 0.9%	Pump reservoir	14 days at 4-22°C and 7 days at 35°C	Am J Hosp Pharm 1992; 49: 619-23
Doxorubicin 1.25 and 0.5 mg/mL in glucose 5%	Pump reservoir	14 days at 4-22°C and 7 days at 35°C	Am J Hosp Pharm 1992; 49: 619-23
Doxorubicin 1.67mg, vincristine 0.036mg/mL	Pump	In NaCl stable for >7 days at 4°C then 4 days at 35°C	Am J Health-Syst Pharm 1996; 53: 1171-3
Doxorubicin 1.67mg, vincristine 0.036mg/mL	Pump PVC	In NaCl stable for >7 days at 4°C then 4 days at 35°C	Am J Health-Syst Pharm 1996; 53: 1171-3
Doxorubicin 2mg/mL in NaCl 0.9%	Pump reservoir	No significant loss after 24 hours at room temperature and 2 days at 5°C	Am J Health-Syst Pharm 1996; 53: 2740-3
Doxorubicin 2mg/mL in NaCl 0.9%	Cassette	>30 days at 30°C	Am J Hosp Pharm 1991; 48: 1976-7
Doxorubicin 4mg/100mL in NaCl 0.9%	Bag	6% loss in 7 days at 4°C	Pharm Weekbl (Sci) 1992; 14: 365-9
Doxorubicin 4mg/100mL in glucose 5%	Bag	10% loss in 7 days at 4°C	Pharm Weekbl (Sci) 1992; 14: 365-9
Doxorubicin and ondansetron.1-2, 0.03-0.3mg/mL	Bag (PVC)	Stable for >48 hours at room temperature	Am J Health-Syst Pharm 1996; 53: 1297-1300
Doxycycline 2mg/mL in NaCl 0.9%	Pump reservoir	24 hours at 5°C 12 hours at 30°C	Am J Hosp Pharm 1995; 52: 70-4
Doxycycline 2mg/mL in water	Pump reservoir	24 hours at 5°C 12 hours at 30°C	Am J Hosp Pharm 1995; 52: 70-4
Doxycycline 100 and 200mg/100 and 250mL in glucose 5%	Bag (PVC)	Stable for 96 hours; 5-9% loss at room temperature and 168 hours at 4°C and 8 hours at room temperature	J Clin Pharm Ther 1994; 19: 317-25
Doxycycline 100 and 200mg/100 and 250mL NaCl 0.9%	Bag (PVC)	Stable for 96 hours; 5-9% loss at room temperature and 168 hours at 4°C and 8 hours at room temperature	J Clin Pharm Ther 1994; 19: 317-25
Doxycycline 100mg and cefmetazole 2g/in glucose 5%	Bag (PVC)	Precipitate in 8 hours at 4°C, <10% loss at room temperature after 96 hours	J Clin Pharm Ther 1994; 19: 317-25
Doxycycline 100mg and cefmetazole 2g/in NaCl 0.9%	Bag (PVC)	Precipitate in 48 hours at 4°C, 10% loss at room temperature after 8 hours	J Clin Pharm Ther 1994; 19: 317-25
Doxycycline 100-200mg and cefmetazole 1g/in glucose 5%	Bag (PVC)	Cefmetazole 72 hours 5-10% degradation; doxycycline stable at room temperature; both <10% degradation after 168 hours at 4°C	J Clin Pharm Ther 1994; 19: 317-25
Doxycycline in glucose 5% or in NaCl 0.9%	Pump (PVC)	48 hours at room temperature, 72 hours in fridge	Trissel
Doxycycline100-200mg and cefmetazole 1g/in NaCl 0.9%	Bag (PVC)	Both stable for 72 hours at room temperature, and for 168 hours at 4°C	J Clin Pharm Ther 1994; 19: 317-25
Droperidol 10mg, morphine 100mg/50mL in NaCl 0.9%	Syringe	14 days at room temperature in light	Hosp Pharm Pract 1992; 2: 597-600
Enoxaparin 120mg/100mL in NaCl 0.9%	Bag (PVC)	At least 48 hours at room temperature	Am J Hosp Pharm 1996; 53: 167-9
Epirubicin 100mg/L in NaCl 0.9% or glucose 5%	Bag	<10% loss in 43 days at 4°C and 25°C in dark	J Clin Pharm Ther 1990; 15: 279-89
Epirubicin 4mg/100mL in NaCl 0.9%	Bag	9% loss in 7 days at 4°C	Pharm Weekbl (Sci) 1992; 14: 365-9
Epirubicin 4mg/100mL in glucose 5%	Bag	No significant loss in 7 days at 4°C	Pharm Weekbl (Sci) 1992; 14: 365-9
Erythromycin 1g/100mL in NaCl 0.9%	Bag	Buffered to pH 7.8, t95% 172 days at 5°C	Int J Pharmaceutics 1992; 80: 7-9
Erythromycin 20mg/mL in NaCl 0.9%	Pump reservoir	24 hours at 5°C and 30°C	Am J Hosp Pharm 1995; 52: 70-4
Erythromycin 20mg/mL in water	Pump reservoir	24 hours at 5°C and 30°C	Am J Hosp Pharm 1995; 52: 70-4

Erythromycin 500mg and 1g/100mL in NaCl 0.9%	Bag	t95% 20 days at 5°C	Int J Pharmaceutics 1992; 80: 7-9
Erythromycin 500mg/100mL in NaCl 0.9%	Bag	Buffered to pH 7.8, t95% 85 days at 5°C	Int J Pharmaceutics 1992; 80: 7-9
Erythromycin in NaCl 0.9%	Pump (PVC)	24 hours at room temperature, 14 days in fridge	Trissel
Erythropoietin 4000u/mL in NaCl 0.9%	Vial	No significant loss after 12 weeks at 5°C and 30°C	Am J Hosp Pharm 1992; 49: 1455-8
Erythropoietin 4000u/mL in NaCl 0.9%	Vial	No significant loss after 12 weeks at 5°C and 30°C	Can J Hosp Pharm 1994; 47: 182
Esmolol 10mg/mL in 500mL sodium bicarbonate 5%	Glass	After 48 hours no significant loss at 5°C, 5% loss at room temperature	Am J Hosp Pharm 1994; 51: 2693-6
Esmolol 10mg/mL in 500mL glucose 5%, and NaCl 0.9%	Bag (PVC)	No significant loss after 7 days at room temperature	Am J Hosp Pharm 1994; 51: 2693-6
Esmolol 10mg/mL in 500mL glucose 5%	Bag (PVC)	No significant loss after 7 days at room temperature	Am J Hosp Pharm 1994; 51: 2693-6
Esmolol 10mg/mL in glucose 5%	Bag (PVC)	No significant loss after 7 days at room temperature	Am J Hosp Pharm 1994; 51: 2693-6
Esmolol 10mg/mL in 500mL NaCl 0.9%	Bag (PVC)	No significant loss after 7 days at room temperature	Am J Hosp Pharm 1994; 51: 2693-6
Esmolol 10mg/mL in 500mL in glucose 5%	Bag (PVC)	No significant loss after 7 days at room temperature	Am J Hosp Pharm 1994; 51: 2693-6
Esmolol 10mg/mL in 500mL compound sodium lactate	Bag (PVC)	No significant loss after 7 days at room temperature	Am J Hosp Pharm 1994; 51: 2693-6
Etoposide 20mg/mL 1:1 in NaCl 0.9%	Syringe	No significant loss after 22 days	Am J Hosp Pharm 1992; 49: 2784-5
Etoposide 400µg/mL in 250mL NaCl 0.9%	Bag	Precipitate in 72 hours at 4°C and room temperature; not recommend, DEHP leached rapidly	Am J Hosp Pharm 1994; 51: 2706-9
Etoposide 400µg/mL in 250mL in NaCl 0.9%	Bag (PVC)	Not recommended; DEHP leached rapidly	Am J Hosp Pharm 1994; 51: 2706-9
Etoposide and ondansetron 100-400, 30-300mg/L	Bag (PVC)	Stable for >48 hours at room temperature	Am J Health-Syst Pharm 1996; 53: 1297-1300
Famotidine 200mg/L in NaCl 0.9%	Bag	No loss in 15 days at 25°C or in 63 days at 5°C	J Clin Pharm Ther 1988; 13: 329-334
Famotidine 200mg/L in glucose 5%	Bag	6% loss in 15 day at 25°C, no loss in 63 days at 5°C	J Clin Pharm Ther 1988; 13: 329-334
Famotidine 200µg/mL in glucose 5%	Bag	Stable for 15 days at room temperature in light	Ann Pharmacother 1993; 27: 422-6
Famotidine 200µg/mL in NaCl 0.9%	Syringe	Stable for 15 days at room temperature in light	Ann Pharmacother 1993; 27: 422-6
Famotidine 20mg and cephazolin 1g/100mL in glucose 5%	Burette	5% loss of cephazolin in 10 hours, 5% loss of famotidine in 24 hours at 4°C, 1 hour at room temperature	Am J Hosp Pharm 1994; 51: 2205-9
Famotidine 2mg/mL in NaCl 0.9%	Syringe	Stable for 8 weeks at -20°C	Am J Hosp Pharm 1990; 47: 2073-4
Famotidine 2mg/mL in glucose 5%	Syringe	Stable for 3 weeks at -20°C	Am J Hosp Pharm 1990; 47: 2073-4
Famotidine 2mg/mL in water, glucose 5%, and NaCl 0.9%	Syringe	No loss in 14 days at 4°C	DICP Ann Pharmacother 1989; 23: 588-90
Famotodine 0.2mg and cefmetazole 5mg/mL in glucose 5%	IV set	168 hours at 4°C and 120 hours at 25°C	Am J Hosp Pharm 1996; 53: 432-3
Fentanyl 20µg/mL in NaCl 0.9%	Pump	>30 days room temperature and 3°C	Am J Hosp Pharm 1990; 47: 1572-4
Fentanyl 2µg/mL and bupivacaine 0.1% in NaCl 0.9%	Bag (PVC)	12 weeks at 8°C and room temperature	Pharm Pract 1995; 5: 21-22
Fentanyl 2µg/mL and bupivacaine 0.1% in NaCl 0.9%	Syringe	12 weeks at 8°C and room temperature	Pharm Pract 1995; 5: 21-22
Fentanyl 4µg/mL and bupivacaine 0.1% in NaCl 0.9%	Bag	12% loss of fentanyl, 9% loss of bupivacaine in 3 days	Br J Anaesth 1992; 68: 414-7
Fentanyl 4µg/mL and bupivacaine 0.1% in NaCl 0.9%	Bag	12% loss in 3 days no further loss in 56 days at room temperature	Br J Anaesth 1992; 68: 414-7
Fentanyl 500µg/500mL in NaCl 0.9%	Bag	>97.8% remaining after 48 hours at room temperature	Am J Hosp Pharm 1990; 47: 1584-7
Fentanyl 500µg/500mL in glucose 5%	Bag	>97.8% remaining after 48 hours at room temperature	Am J Hosp Pharm 1990; 47: 1584-7
Fentanyl and bupivacaine in NaCl 0.9%	Cassette	30 days at 23°C	Am J Hosp Pharm 1990; 47: 2037-40
Flucloxacillin 25 and 50mg/mL in water	Syringe	3 or 7 days in fridge, use within 24 hours at room temperature	Pharm J 1992; 248(Suppl): HS20-1
Flucloxacillin 250mg/1.8mL in water 0.16mL	Syringe	7 days in fridge	Hosp Pharm Pract 1992; 2: 285-9
Flucloxacillin 2 and 1g/100mL in NaCl 0.9%	Bag	10% loss after 28 days in fridge, 21day shelf-life	Hosp Pharm Pract 1993; 3: 553-6
Flucloxacillin 500mg/100mL in NaCl 0.9%	Bag	8% loss after 35 days in fridge, 21day shelf-life	Hosp Pharm Pract 1993; 3: 553-6
Flucloxacillin 5mg/mL in NaCl 0.9%	Bag	3 days in fridge, use within 24 hours at room temperature	Pharm J 1992; 248(Suppl): HS20-1
Fluconazole 1mg/mL in glucose 5%	Vial	No significant loss at 25°C in light after 24 hours	Am J Hosp Pharm 1993; 50: 1186-7
Fluconazole 1mg/mL in KCl in glucose 5%	Vial	No significant loss at 25°C in light after 72 hours	Am J Hosp Pharm 1993; 50: 1186-7
Fluconazole 1mg/mL in compound sodium lactate	Vial	No significant loss at 25°C in light after 24 hours	Am J Hosp Pharm 1993; 50: 1186-7
Flumazenil 1mg in 50mL glucose 5%	Bag	No loss in 24 hours at 23°C in light	Am J Hosp Pharm 1993; 50: 1907-12
Flumazenil/aminophylline 1/2mg/50mLin glucose 5%	Bag	No loss in 24 hours at 23°C in light	Am J Hosp Pharm 1993; 50: 1907-12
Flumazenil/cimetidine 1/2.4mg/50mL in glucose 5%	Bag	No loss in 24 hours at 23°C in light	Am J Hosp Pharm 1993; 50: 1907-12
Flumazenil/dobutamine 1/2mg/50mL in glucose 5%	Bag	No loss in 24 hours at 23°C in light	Am J Hosp Pharm 1993; 50: 1907-12
Flumazenil/dopamine 1/3.2mg/50mL in glucose 5%	Bag	5% loss of flumazenil in 12 hours at 23°C in light	Am J Hosp Pharm 1993; 50: 1907-12

Flumazenil/famotidine 1/0.08mg/50mL in glucose 5%	Bag	No loss in 24 hours at 23°C in light	Am J Hosp Pharm 1993; 50: 1907-12
Flumazenil/heparin sodium 1mg/50u/50mL in glucose 5%	Bag	No loss of f in 24 hours at 23°C in light	Am J Hosp Pharm 1993; 50: 1907-12
Flumazenil/lignocaine hydrochloride 1/4mg/50mL in glucose 5%	Bag	No loss in 24 hours at 23°C in light	Am J Hosp Pharm 1993; 50: 1907-12
Flumazenil/procainamide 1/4mg/50mL in glucose 5%	Bag	No loss in 24 hours at 23°C in light	Am J Hosp Pharm 1993; 50: 1907-12
Flumazenil/ranitidine 1/0.3mg/50mL in glucose 5%	Bag	No loss in 24 hours at 23°C in light	Am J Hosp Pharm 1993; 50: 1907-12
Fluorouracil 1 or 10mg/mL in NaCl 0.9%	Bag PVC	Stable for 14 days at 21°C and 4°C	J Pharm Biomed Anal 1996; 14: 395-9
Fluorouracil 1 or 10mg/mL in glucose 5%	Bag PVC	Stable for 14 days at 21°C and 4°C	J Pharm Biomed Anal 1996; 14: 395-9
Fluorouracil 10 and 50mg/mL in NaCl 0.9%	Pump reservoir	28 days at 4-35°C	Am J Hosp Pharm 1992; 49: 619-23
Fluorouracil 10 and 50mg/mL in glucose 5%	Pump reservoir	28 days at 4-35°C	Am J Hosp Pharm 1992; 49: 619-23
Fluorouracil 1g and carboplatin 100mg in glucose 5%	Bag	10% loss in 5 hours at 25°C	J Clin Pharm Ther 1994; 19: 127-33
Fluorouracil 1g and carboplatin 100mg in glucose 5%	Bag	Stable for 48 hours at room temperature	J Clin Pharm Ther 1994; 19: 127-33
Fluorouracil 1g and carboplatin 100mg/L in glucose 5%	Bag	16% loss of carboplatin at room temperature	J Clin Pharm Ther 1994; 19: 127-33
Fluorouracil 1g and carboplatin 100mg/L in glucose 5%	Bag	2.8% loss of carboplatin at room temperature	J Clin Pharm Ther 1994; 19: 127-33
Fluorouracil 250mg and metoclopramide 10mg	IV set	In glucose, 5% loss after 4 hours at room temperature and 120 hours at 4°C	Am J Hosp Pharm 1996; 53: 98-9
Fluorouracil 500mg and heparin 20000u/20.8mL	Syringe	No significant loss after 14 days at 4°C and 7 days at room temperature, and at 37°C	J Clin Pharm Ther 1994; 19: 127-33
Fluorouracil 50mg/mL	Pump (EVA)	Stable for 14 days at 33°C but precipitates in 3 days at 4°C	J Pharm Biomed Anal 1996; 14: 395-9
Fluorouracil 50mg/mL	Pump (PVC)	Stable for 14 days at 33°C but precipitates in 5 days at 4°C	J Pharm Biomed Anal 1996; 14: 395-9
Fluorouracil 5mg/mL in NaCl 0.9%	Pump reservoir	No significant loss after 24 hours at room temperature	Am J Health-Syst Pharm 1996; 53: 2740-3
Foscarnet sodium 12mg/mL in NaCl 0.9%	Bag	Stable for 30 days at 5 and 25°C	Am J Hosp Pharm 1994; 51: 88-90
Foscarnet undiluted or up to 1mg/mL in NaCl 0.9%	Pump (PVC)	24 hours at room temperature, 35 days at 4°C	J Clin Pharm Ther 1989; 14: 451-6
Frusemide 10mg/mL	Syringe	2 months at room temperature and 4°C	Pharm J 1992; 248(Suppl): HS40-1
Frusemide 2mg/mL in glucose 5% and 10%	Bag	24 hours; no chemical degradation	Hosp Pharm Pract 1991; 1: 191-5
Frusemide 5mg and ciprofloxacin 2mg/mL	Y-site	Incompatible	Ann Pharmacother 1993; 27: 704-7
Frusemide and labetalol	Line	Incompatible	Am J Hosp Pharm 1993; 50: 2521-2
Ganciclovir 100mg/100mL in NaCl 0.9%	Bag	Stable for 35 days at 5°C and 25°C	Am J Hosp Pharm 1992; 49: 116-8
Ganciclovir 100mg/100mL in glucose 5%	Bag	Stable for 35 days at 5°C and 25°C	Am J Hosp Pharm 1992; 49: 116-8
Ganciclovir 1, 5 and 10mg/mL in glucose 5%	Bag	No significant loss at 4°C after 35 days	Am J Hosp Pharm 1991; 48: 2641-3
Ganciclovir 2 and 4mg/mL in 100mL NaCl 0.9%	Bag	5 weeks at 4°C	Pharm J 1992; 248(Suppl): HS40-1
Ganciclovir 500mg/100mL in NaCl 0.9%	Bag	Stable for 35 days at 5°C and 25°C	Am J Hosp Pharm 1992; 49: 116-8
Ganciclovir 500mg/100mL in glucose 5%	Bag	Stable for 35 days at 5°C and 25°C	Am J Hosp Pharm 1992; 49: 116-8
Ganciclovir 5mg/mL in NaCl 0.9%	Pump reservoir	4% loss after 24 hours at 25°C and 6% after 5 days at 5°C	Am J Health-Syst Pharm 1996; 53: 2740-3
Ganciclovir 5.8mg/mL in NaCl 0.9%	Pump	No significant degradation after 12 hours at 25°C and 10 days at 4°C	Am J Hosp Pharm 1994; 51: 1348-9
Ganciclovir in glucose 5% or in NaCl 0.9%	Pump (PVC)	35 days at room temperature, 35 days in fridge	Trissel
Gentamicin 0.8mg/mL in NaCl 0.9%	Pump reservoir	No significant loss after 24 hours at 25°C	Am J Health-Syst Pharm 1996; 53: 2740-3
Gentamicin 10mg/mL	Syringe	Stable for 7 days	Hosp Pharm Pract 1991; 1: 243-252
Gentamicin 120mg in glucose 5% and in NaCl 0.9%	Bag	Stable for 48 hours at room temperature and 4°C	Am J Hosp Pharm 1991; 48: 2166-71
Gentamicin 60 and 120mg/20mL in glucose 10%	Vial	No significant degradation after 30 days	Am J Hosp Pharm 1994; 51: 518-9
Gentamicin in glucose 5% or in NaCl 0.9%	Pump (PVC)	24 hours at room temperature, 96 hours in fridge	Trissel
Gentamicin and ciprofloxacin 120/200mg in 100mL NaCl 0.9%	Bag	Both stable for 48 hours at room temperature and 4°C	Am J Hosp Pharm 1991; 48: 2166-71
Gentamicin and ciprofloxacin 120/200mg in 100mL glucose 5%	Bag	Both stable for 48 hours at room temperature and 4°C	Am J Hosp Pharm 1991; 48: 2166-71
Glyceryl trinitrate 25mg/25mL in NaCl 0.9%	Syringe	5% loss in 7 days, 10% in 3 weeks at 4°C; 10% loss after 7 days and 15% after 3 weeks at room temperature	Hosp Pharm Pract 1992; 2: 137-141
Glyceryl trinitrate 25mg/25mL in glucose 5%	Syringe	5% loss in 7 days, 10% in 3 weeks at 4°C; 8% loss in 7 days and 10% after 2 weeks at room temperature	Hosp Pharm Pract 1992; 2: 137-141
Granisetron 0.02mg/mL in NaCl 0.9%	Pump	Stable for 7 days at 4°C	Am J Health-Syst Pharm 1995; 52: 1541-3
Granisetron 0.02mg/mL in glucose 5%	Pump	Stable for 14 days at 4°C	Am J Health-Syst Pharm 1995; 52: 1541-3
Granisetron 0.05-0.1mg/mL in NaCl or in glucose 5%	Syringe	No significant loss after 14 days at 5°C and 24°C	Am J Health-Syst Pharm 1996; 53: 2744-6

Granisetron 1mg with many other drugs	Y-site	See reference for details	Am J Hosp Pharm 1996; 53: 294-303
Granisetron 1mg/50mL in NaCl 0.9%	Bag (PVC)	At least 24 hours at room temperature	Am J Hosp Pharm 1996; 53: 294-303
Granisetron 1mg/50mL in glucose 5%	Bag (PVC)	At least 24 hours at room temperature	Am J Hosp Pharm 1996; 53: 294-303
Granisetron 1mg/5mL in NaCl 0.9%	Syringe	At least 24 hours at room temperature	Am J Hosp Pharm 1996; 53: 294-303
Granisetron 1mg/5mL in glucose 5%	Syringe	At least 24 hours at room temperature	Am J Hosp Pharm 1996; 53: 294-303
Granisetron and dexamethasone in NaCl 0.9%	Bag (PVC)	Stable for 14 days at room temperature or 4°C	Am J Health-Syst Pharm 1996; 53: 1174-6
Granisetron and dexamethasone in glucose 5%	Bag (PVC)	Stable for 14 days at room temperature or 4°C	Am J Health-Syst Pharm 1996; 53: 1174-6
Granisetron, dexamethasone and methylprednisolone		See reference for details	J Pharm Sci 84: 267-8
Heparin 1u and ciprofloxacin 2mg/mL	Y-site	Incompatible	Ann Pharmacother 1993; 27: 704-7
Heparin and fluorouracil 500mg/20.8mL	Syringe	No significant loss after 14 days at 4°C and 7 days at room temperature	J Clin Pharm Ther 1994; 19: 127-33
Hydrocortisone sodium succinate 100mg in 100mL NaCl 0.9%	Bag	10% degradation after 3 days at room temperature and 26 days at 4°C	Pharm J 1992; 248(Suppl): HS40-1
Hydrocortisone sodium succinate 100mg/100mL in glucose 5%	Bag	10% degradation after 3 days at room temperature and 56 days at 4°C	Pharm J 1992; 248(Suppl): HS40-1
Hydrocortisone sodium succinate 100mg/2mL in water	Syringe	10% degradation after 3 days at room temperature and 42 days at 4°C	Pharm J 1992; 248(Suppl): HS40-1
Hydromorphone 0.5mg and ondansetron 0.1 and 1mg	Glass	>31 days at 4 and 22°C and 7 days at 32°C in NaCl 0.9%	Am J Hosp Pharm 1994; 51: 2138-42
Hydromorphone/dimethylhydrinate	Vial	See reference for details	Can J Hosp Pharm 1993; 46: 61-65
Hydromorphone/lorazepam/prochlorperazine	Vial	See reference for details	Can J Hosp Pharm 1993; 46: 61-65
Ifosfamide 10-80mg/mL in NaCl 0.9%	Cassette	8 days at room temperature	Am J Hosp Pharm 1992; 49: 1137-9
Ifosfamide 50mg in NaCl 0.9%	Syringe	21 days at 4°C and room temperature	Pharm J 1992; 248(Suppl): HS40-1
Imipenem/cilastatin 5mg/mL in NaCl 0.9%	Pump reservoir	No significant loss after 4 hours at 25°C and 24 hours at 5°C:	Am J Health-Syst Pharm 1996; 53: 2740-3
Imipenem/cilastatin 5mg/mL in glucose 5%	Pump reservoir	No significant loss after 4 hours at 25°C and 24 hours at 5°C	Am J Health-Syst Pharm 1996; 53: 2740-3
Imipenem/cilastatin in glucose 5% or NaCl 0.9%	Pump (PVC)	10 hours at room temperature, 48 hours in fridge; glucose 4 hours at room temperature, 24 hours fridge	Trissel
Imipenem/cilastatin 2.5-5g/L in NaCl 0.9%	Bottle	6-8% loss in 9 hours at 25°C, 7% in 48 hours	Am J Hosp Pharm 1986; 43: 2803-9
Imipenem/cilastatin 2.5-5g/L in glucose 5%	Bottle	5-6% loss in 6 hours at 25°C, 6% in 24 hours and 11% in 48 hours at 4°C	Am J Hosp Pharm 1986; 43: 2803-9
Immunoglobulin in glucose 5%	Bag	Stable for 24 hours at room temperature	Ann Pharmacother 1994; 28: 1014-7
Insulin (soluble, isophane, combined)	Syringe	No significant loss at room temperature and 4°C after 28 days	Am J Hosp Pharm 1991; 48: 2631-4
Intoplicine 0.1 and 1mg/mL in NaCl 0.9%	Bottle	No significant loss after 7 days at room temperature or 4°C	J Pharm Biomed Anal 1993; 11: 1353-6
Intoplicine 0.1 and 1mg/mL in glucose 5%	Bottle	No significant loss after 7 days at room temperature or 4°C	J Pharm Biomed Anal 1993; 11: 1353-6
Isosorbide 40mg/540mL in NaCl 0.9%	Bag	>70% loss in 15-30 minutes due to adsorption	J Clin Hosp Pharm 1981; 6: 209
Ketamine 20mg, morphine 1mg/mL in NaCl 0.9%	Syringe	No significant degradation in 4 days	Hosp Pharm Pract 1994; 4: 57-58
Ketamine 20mg/mL in NaCl 0.9%	Syringe	No significant degradation in 4 days	Hosp Pharm Pract 1994; 4: 57-8
Labetalol and frusemide	Line	Incompatible	Am J Hosp Pharm1993; 50: 2521-2
Levofloxacin 0.5 and 5mg/mL in NaCl 0.9%	Bag (PVC)	No significant degradation after 3 days at 25°C and 14 days at 5°C	Am J Health-Syst Pharm 1996; 53: 2309-13
Levofloxacin 0.5 and 5mg/mL in 10 diluents	Bag (PVC)	No significant degradation at 5°C and 25°C for 14 and 3 days. Precipitate at -20°C for 2 diluents	Am J Health-Syst Pharm 1996; 53: 2309-13
Levofloxacin 0.5 and 5mg/mL in glucose 5%	Bag (PVC)	No significant degradation after 3 days at 25°C and 14 days at 5°C	Am J Health-Syst Pharm 1996; 53: 2309-13
Lignocaine 0.6mg and nafcillin 20mg/mL in glucose 5%	Bag (PVC)	48 hours at room temperature	Am J Hosp Pharm 1995; 52: 521-3
Lignocaine 0.6mg and nafcillin 20mg/mL in NaCl	Bag	48 hours at room temperature	Am J Hosp Pharm 1995; 52: 521-3
Lignocaine 1%	Syringe	6 months at room temperature	Hosp Pharm Pract 1992; 2: 633-67
Lignocaine and ranitidine in NaCl 0.9%	Bag (PVC)	Stable for 48 hours	Am J Hosp Pharm 1994; 51: 1802-7
Lorazepam/dexamphetamine/ondansetron/in glucose 5%	Bag	Lorazepam loss >10% in 4 hours	Am J Hosp Pharm 1993; 50: 1410-4
Lorazepam/dexamphetamine/ondansetron in NaCl 0.9%	Bag	Lorazepam loss >10% in 4 hours	Am J Hosp Pharm 1993; 50: 1410-4
Lorazepam 0.08 and 0.5mg/mL in glucose 5% and NaCl	Bag (PVC)	Loss of >10% in 1 hour at room temperature and 4°C	Ann Pharmacother 1996; 30: 343-6

Lorazepam 0.1mg/mL in NaCl 0.9%	Bag	Stable for 7 days at 4°C and 24°C	Am J Hosp Pharm 1994; 51: 368-72
Lorazepam 0.1mg/mL in NaCl 0.9%	Bag PVC	Stable for 7 days at 4°C, 8 hours at 24°C due to sorption	Am J Hosp Pharm 1994; 51: 368-72
Lorazepam 0.1mg/mL in glucose 5%	Bag	Stable for 7 days at 4°C and 24°C	Am J Hosp Pharm 1994; 51: 368-72
Lorazepam 0.1mg/mL in glucose 5%	Bag PVC	Stable for 7 days at 4°C, 8 hours at 24°C due to sorption	Am J Hosp Pharm 1994; 51: 368-72
Lorazepam 0.1mg/mL in compound sodium lactate	Bag	Stable for 7 days at 4°C and 24°C	Am J Hosp Pharm 1994; 51: 368-72
Lorazepam 0.1mg/mL in compound sodium lactate	Bag PVC	Stable for 24 hours at 4°C, <8 hours at 24°C	Am J Hosp Pharm 1994; 51: 368-72
Lorazepam/metoclopramide/dexamethasone/in NaCl	Pump	Lorazepam 15% loss in 24 hours, others stable for 15 days	Am J Hosp Pharm 1994; 51: 514-7
Melphalan 0.2mg/mL in 50mL NaCl 0.9%	Bag (PVC)	Stable for 6 hours at 4°C, 3 hours at room temperature	Am J Hosp Pharm 1994; 51: 2701-4
Melphalan 0.2mg/mL in 50mL NaCl 0.9%	Bag (PVC)	Stable for 48 hours at 4°C, 6 hours at room temperature	Am J Hosp Pharm 1994; 51: 2701-4
Meropenem 1-20mg/mL in NaCl 0.9%	Bag	48 hours at 4°C, 8 hours at room temperature	ABPI. Data sheet 1996-7
Meropenem 1-20mg/mL in glucose 5% and NaCl 0.9%	Bag	14 hours at 4°C, 3 hours at room temperature	ABPI. Data sheet 1996-7
Meropenem 1 and 20mg/mL in glucose 5%	Bag (PVC)	10% degradation at 4°C in 18 hours and 4% in 4 hours at room temperature	Am J Health-Syst Pharm 1997; 54: 412-21
Meropenem 1 and 20mg/mL in water and NaCl 0.9%	Bag (PVC)	5% degradation at 4°C in 48 hours and 10% in 24 hours at room temperature	Am J Health-Syst Pharm 1997; 54: 412-21
Methicillin in glucose 5% or NaCl 0.9%	Pump (PVC)	24 hours at room temperature, 4 days in fridge	Trissel
Methotrexate 22.5mg/100mL or 12g/500mL	Bag (PVC)	No significant loss after 30 days at 4°C in NaCl 0.9% or in glucose 5%	Int J Pharmaceutics 1994; 105: 83-87
Methotrexate 2.5mg/mL	Syringe	Stable for at least 7 days at 4°C and room temperature	Int J Pharmaceutics 1996; 128: 283-6
Methotrexate 50mg/mL	Syringe	Stable for 8 months at room temperature	Int J Pharmaceutics 1988; 45: 237-44 t
Methotrexate and ondansetron 5-6, 0.03-0.3mg/mL	Bag (PVC)	Stable for >48 hours at room temperature	Am J Health-Syst Pharm 1996; 53: 1297-1300
Methylprednisolone sodium succinate 4mg/mL in water	Glass	5% loss in 7 days, 16% in 14 days at 4°C, 10% in 24 hours at 22°C	Am J Hosp Pharm 1994; 51: 2157-59
Methylprednisolone and ranitidine in NaCl 0.9%	Bag (PVC)	Stable for 48 hours	Am J Hosp Pharm 1994; 51: 1802-7
Metoclopramide 10mg and fluorouracil 250mg	IV set	In glucose 5% 4 hours at room temperature and 120 hours at 4°C	Am J Hosp Pharm 1996; 53: 98-9
Metoclopramide 30mg and morphine 60mg/60mL	Infusor	In glucose 5%, 4 months at 4°C, 14 days at room temperature	Pharm J 1995; 254: 153-5
Metoclopramide 30mg and morphine 60mg/60mL	Syringe	In NaCl 0.9%, at least 4 months at 4°C, 14 days at room temperature	Pharm J 1995; 254: 153-5
Metoclopramide 50mg and morphine 100mg/100mL	Bag	In NaCl 0.9%, at least 4 months at 4°C, 14 days at room temperature	Pharm J 1995; 254: 153-5
Metoclopramide/dexamethasone/lorazepam in NaCl 0.9%	Pump	Lorazepam 15% loss in 24 hours, others stable for 15 days	Am J Hosp Pharm 1994; 51: 514-7
Metoprolol tartrate 0.4mg/mL in NaCl 0.9%	Bag	<5% loss in 36 hours at room temperature	Am J Hosp Pharm 1993; 50: 950-2
Metoprolol tartrate 0.4mg/mL in glucose 5%	Bag	<5% loss in 36 hours at room temperature	Am J Hosp Pharm 1993; 50: 950-2
Metronidazole 25mg/5mL	Syringe	Stable for 3 months in fridge	Hosp Pharm Pract 1991; 1: 243-252
Metronidazole 5mg/5mL in glucose 5%	Syringe	Stable for 3 months in fridge	Hosp Pharm Pract 1991; 1: 243-252
Metronidazole in glucose 5% or in NaCl 0.9%	Pump (PVC)	24 hours at room temperature	Trissel
Metronidazole 0.5% and cefuroxime 750mg, 1.5g	Bag	Shelf-life of 1 month	Pharm Pract 1995; 5: 100-106
Metronidazole 0.5% and ciprofloxacin 200mg/100mL	Bag	Both stable for 48 hours at room temperature and 4°C	Am J Hosp Pharm 1991; 48: 2166-71
Metronidazole 500mg and ceftazidime 1g/100mL	Bag (PVC)	No significant loss of either at 8°C after 72 hours	Am J Hosp Pharm 1995; 52: 2568-70
Metronidazole 500mg and ceftizoxime 1g/100mL	Bag (PVC)	No significant loss of either at 8°C after 72 hours	Am J Hosp Pharm 1995; 52: 2568-70
Metronidazole 500mg and ceftriaxone 1g/100mL	Bag (PVC)	No significant loss of either at 8°C after 72 hours	Am J Hosp Pharm 1995; 52: 2568-70
Metronidazole 500mg/cefuroxime 750mg	Bag	7 days at 4°C	J Clin Pharm Ther 1990; 15: 187-96
Mezlocillin 10g/L in NaCl 0.9%	Bag	2% loss in 4 days and 9% in 7 days at 25°C, 2% loss in 36 days at 5°C	J Pharm Sci 1983; 72: 1479-81
Mezlocillin 10g/L in glucose 5%	Bag	4% loss in 4 days and 10% in 7 days at 25°C, 3% loss in 36 days at 5°C	J Pharm Sci 1983; 72: 1479-81
Mezlocillin 20mg/mL in glucose 5%	Pump reservoir	5% loss after 48 hours at 25°C and 7 days at 5°C	Am J Health-Syst Pharm 1996; 53: 2740-3
Mezlocillin in glucose 5% or in NaCl 0.9%	Pump (PVC)	48 hours at room temperature, 7 days in fridge	Trissel
Miconazole 2.42mg/mL in glucose 5% or in NaCl 0.9%	Bag (PVC)	Stable for 24 hours at room temperature and 4°C	J Pharm Biomed Anal 1995; 13: 1363-72
Midazolam 0.5mg/mL in NaCl 0.9%	Bag	Stable for at least 30 days in fridge and at room temperature	Am J Hosp Pharm 1993; 50: 2379-81
Midazolam 0.5mg/mL in glucose 5%	Bag	Stable for at least 30 days in fridge and at room temperature	Am J Hosp Pharm 1993; 50: 2379-81

Midazolam 10mg, diamorphine 10mg/15mL in water	Syringe	Stable for 14 days at room temperature	Int J Pharm Pract 1994; 3: 57-9
Midazolam 1mg/mL in NaCl 0.9%	Bag (PVC)	5% loss after 10 days at 23°C in light and dark	Am J Health-Syst Pharm 1995; 52: 2018-20
Midazolam 1mg/mL in NaCl 0.9%	Bag	4-6% loss in 49 days at 20°C and 4°C	Aust J Hosp Pharm 1993; 23: 260-2
Midazolam 75mg, diamorphine 500mg/15mL in water	Syringe	Stable for 14 days at room temperature	Int J Pharm Pract 1994; 3: 57-9
Minocycline hydrochloride 0.1mg/mL in NaCl 0.9%	Bag	2% loss in 7 days at 4°C, 8% at room temperature in 7 days	Am J Hosp Pharm 1993; 50: 698-701
Minocycline hydrochloride 0.1mg/mL in glucose 5%	Bag	2% loss in 7 days at 4°C, 8% at room temperature in 7 days	Am J Hosp Pharm 1993; 50: 698-701
Mitomycin 400mg/L in glucose 5%	Bag	10% loss in 1-2 hours at room temperature	Am J Hosp Pharm 1981; 38: 1914-8
Mitomycin 50mg/L in NaCl 0.9%	Bag	10% loss in 5 days at 25°C	Arch Pharm Chemi (Sci) 1985: 58-66
Mitomycin 50mg/L in NaCl 0.9%	Bag	10% loss in 12 hours at 5°C violet colour in 4 hours	Am J Hosp Pharm 1985; 42: 1750-4
Mitomycin 50mg/L in glucose 5%	Bag	10% loss in 2.6 hours at room temperature	Arch Pharm Chemi (Sci) 1985: 58-66
Mitozantrone 0.05mg and etoposide 0.5mg/mL		No loss in 24 hours at room temperature in dark in NaCl 0.9%	Acta Pharm Nord 1991; 3: 251
Mitozantrone 0.1mg and etoposide 1mg		No loss in 24 hours at room temperature in dark	Acta Pharm Nord 1991; 3: 251
Molsidomine 80µg/mL in NaCl 0.9%	Bag	Half-life of 20 minutes when exposed to light	J Pharm Pharmacol 1993; 45: 486-8
Morphine 100mg, droperidol 10mg/50mL in NaCl	Syringe	14 days at room temperature in light	Hosp Pharm Pract 1992; 2: 597-600
Morphine 100mg, metoclopramide 50mg/100mL	Bag	In NaCl 0.9%, at least 4 months at 4°C, 14 days at room temperature	Pharm J 1995; 254: 153-5
Morphine 100mg/50mL in NaCl 0.9%	Syringe	Stable for 6 weeks at room temperature	Pharm J 1992; 248(Suppl): HS24-6
Morphine 100mg/50mL in NaCl 0.9%	Syringe	With sodium metabisulphite 15% degradation in 6 weeks	Pharm J 1992; 248(Suppl): HS24-6
Morphine 1mg and ondansetron 0.1and 1mg/mL	Glass	>31 days at 4 and 22°C and 7 days at 32°C in NaCl 0.9%	Am J Hosp Pharm 1994; 51: 2138-42
Morphine 1mg/mL in NaCl 0.9%	Syringe	No significant degradation in 4 days	Hosp Pharm Pract 1994; 4: 57-8
Morphine 240mg, ketamine 100mg/10mL in NaCl 0.9%	Syringe	8 days room temperature and fridge	Aust J Hosp Pharm 1995; 5: 352
Morphine 2mg/mL in NaCl 0.9%	Syringe	<5% loss in 6 weeks	Int J Pharm Pract 1993; 2: 39-43
Morphine 50mg, morphine 10mg/50mL in NaCl 0.9%	Pump	No significant degradation after 30 days at 37°C	Int J Pharmaceutics 1995; 118: 181-9
Morphine 60mg, metoclopramide 30mg/60mL	Syringe	In NaCl 0.9%, at least 4 months at 4°C, 14 days at room temperature	Pharm J 1995; 254: 153-5
Morphine 60mg, metoclopramide 30mg/60mL	Infusor	In glucose 5%, 4 months at 4°C, 14 days at room temperature	Pharm J 1995; 254: 153-5
Morphine hydrochloride 0.5, 1.5 and 2.5mg/mL in NaCl 0.9%	Cassette	No loss for 60 days at 32°C	Pharm Weekbl (Sci) 1992; 14: 23-6
Morphine 0.5-30mg/mL in NaCl 0.9%	Bag	14 days at 5°C and 37°C	Am J Hosp Pharm 1990; 47: 2040-2
Morphine and baclofen	Pump	Stable for >30 days at 37°C	Aust J Hosp Pharm 1992; 22: 258
Morphine and midazolam or haloperidol		See reference for details	Can J Hosp Pharm 1995; 48: 155-6
Morphine and ketamine 1 and 20mg/mL in NaCl 0.9%	Syringe	No significant degradation in 4 days	Hosp Pharm Pract 1994; 4: 57-8
Moxalactam 10mg/mL in NaCl 0.9%	Bag	3% loss in 24 hours at 24°C, 5% in 11 days at 5°C	Am J Intravenous Ther 1983: 20-29
Moxalactam 10mg/mL in glucose 5%	Bag	6% loss in 24 hours at 24°C, 6% in 11 days at 5°C	Am J Intravenous Ther 1983: 20-29
Moxalactam 20mg/mL in NaCl 0.9%	Bag	6-8% loss in 24 hours at 25°C, 3-4% in 96 hours at 5°C	Am J Hosp Pharm 1982; 39: 1495-8
Moxalactam 20mg/mL in glucose 5%	Bag	6-8% loss in 24 hours at 25°C, 1-6% in 96 hours at 5°C	Am J Hosp Pharm 1982; 39: 1495-8
Mustine 1mg/mL in water or in NaCl 0.9%	Syringe	8-10% loss in 6 hours at 22°C, 4-6% at 6 hours at 4°C	Br J Parenter Ther 1986; 7: 86-7
Mustine 20mg/L in NaCl 0.9%	Bag	10% loss in 3 hours at 22°C, 10% loss in 4 hours at 4°C	Br J Parenter Ther 1986; 7: 86-7
Mustine 20mg/L in glucose 5%	Bag	10% loss in 5 hours at 22°C, 4% loss in 6 hours at 4°C	Br J Parenter Ther 1986; 7: 86-7
Nafcillin 20mg and lignocaine 0.6mg/mL in glucose 5%	Bag (PVC)	48 hours at room temperature	Am J Hosp Pharm 1995; 52: 521-3
Nafcillin 20mg and lignocaine 0.6mg/mL in NaCl 0.9%	Bag	48 hours at room temperature	Am J Hosp Pharm 1995; 52: 521-3
Nafcillin 20mg/mL in NaCl 0.9%	Pump reservoir	2% loss after 24 hours at 25°C and none after 4 days at 5°C	Am J Health-Syst Pharm 1996; 53: 2740-3
Nafcillin 20mg/mL in glucose 5%	Pump reservoir	3% loss after 24 hours at 25°C and 2% after 4 days at 5°C	Am J Health-Syst Pharm 1996; 53: 2740-3
Nafcillin 80mg/mL in NaCl 0.9%	Pump reservoir	48 hours at 5°C and 30°C	Am J Hosp Pharm 1995; 52: 70-4
Nafcillin 80mg/mL in water	Pump reservoir	48 hours at 5°C and 30°C	Am J Hosp Pharm 1995; 52: 70-4
Nafcillin in glucose 5% or in NaCl 0.9%	Pump (PVC)	24 hours at room temperature, 96 hours in fridge	Trissel
Netilmicin 15mg/1.5mL	Syringe	30 days at 4°C	Pharm J 1992; 248(Suppl): HS40-1
Nicardipine 0.05-0.5mg/mL in various fluids	Bag	See reference for details	Am J Health-Syst Pharm 1996; 53: 1701-5
Nicardipine 0.05-0.5mg/mL in NaCl 0.9%	Bag	5% loss in 7 days at room temperature	Am J Health-Syst Pharm 1996; 53: 1701-5

Nicardipine 0.05-0.5mg/mL in glucose 5%	Bag	10% loss in 7 days at room temperature	Am J Health-Syst Pharm 1996; 53: 1701-5
Nitroglycerin 10mg/100mL in NaCl 0.9%	Bag	No significant loss in 120 hours at room temperature	Int J Pharmaceutics 1994; 110: 197-201
Nitroglycerin 10mg/100mL in NaCl 0.9%	Bag (PVC)	60% loss in 20 hours at room temperature	Int J Pharmaceutics 1994; 110: 197-201
Nitroglycerin 5mg/mL	Syringe	Stable for at least 23 hours at 25°C	Am J Hosp Pharm1993; 50: 2561-3
Nitroglycerin 5mg/mL	Syringe	Stable for at least 23 hours at 25°C	Am J Hosp Pharm1993; 50: 2561-3
Nitroglycerin 5mg/mL	Syringe	Stable for at least 23 hours at 25°C	Am J Hosp Pharm1993; 50: 2561-3
Noradrenaline and ranitidine in NaCl 0.9%	Bag (PVC)	Stable for 48 hours	Am J Hosp Pharm 1994; 51: 1802-7
Octreotide 0.2mg/mL	Syringe	Stable for 29 days at 3°C	Am J Hosp Pharm 1993; 50: 2356-8
Octreotide 200µg/mL	Syringe	5% loss after 60 days at 5°C and -20°C	Am J Health-Syst Pharm 1995; 52: 1910-1
Ofloxacin 0.4 and 4mg/mL in NaCl 0.9%	Bag	No significant loss at 24°C after 3 days or 5°C after 14 days	Am J Hosp Pharm 1992; 49: 2756-2760
Ofloxacin 0.4 and 4mg/mL in glucose 5%	Bag	No significant loss at 24°C after 3 days or 5°C after 14 days	Am J Hosp Pharm 1992; 49: 2756-2760
Ofloxacin 0.4 and 4mg/mL in NaCl 0.9% and in glucose 5%	Bag	No significant loss at 24°C after 3 days or 5°C after 14 days	Am J Hosp Pharm 1992; 49: 2756-2760
Ofloxacin 0.4 and 4mg/mL in various fluids	Bag	No significant loss at 24°C after 3 days or 5°C after 14 days	Am J Hosp Pharm 1992; 49: 2756-2760
Ofloxacin 0.8mg/mL in 250mL of NaCl 0.9%	Bag	No significant loss at room temperature in light after 6 hours	Int J Pharmaceutics 1993; 89: 125-131
Ofloxacin 0.8mg/mL in 250mL of glucose 5%	Bag	No significant loss at room temperature in light after 6 hours	Int J Pharmaceutics 1993; 89: 125-131
Ondansetron 0.03 and 0.3mg/mL in NaCl 0.9%	Pump	No significant loss after 14 days at 4°C	Am J Hosp Pharm 1993; 50: 1918-20
Ondansetron 0.03 and 0.3mg/mL in glucose 5%	Pump	No significant loss after 14 days at 4°C	Am J Hosp Pharm 1993; 50: 1918-20
Ondansetron 0.03 and 0.3mg/mL in glucose 5% and in NaCl 0.9%	Bag	>48 hours at 25°C, 14 days at 5°C, 3 months at -20°C	Am J Hosp Pharm 1992; 49: 2223-5
Ondansetron 0.08mg/mL in NaCl 0.9%	Bag	<5% degradation after 120 days at 4°C and -20°C	Eur J Hosp Pharm 1994; 4: 12-13
Ondansetron 80mg/L in glucose 5% or NaCl 0.9%	Syringe	Stable for 7 days at room temperature or 4°C	Eur J Cancer Clin Oncol 1989: 67-9
Ondansetron 0.05mg and cyclophosphamide 0.3mg	Bag (PVC)	8 days at 4°C or 4 days at room temperature	Am J Hosp Pharm 1995; 52: 514-6
Ondansetron 0.4mg and cyclophosphamide 2mg/mL	Bag (PVC)	8 days at 4°C or 4 days at room temperature	Am J Hosp Pharm 1995; 52: 514-6
Ondansetron 16-80mg/L in NaCl 0.9%	Bag	Stable for 7 days at room temperature or 4°C	Eur J Cancer Clin Oncol 1989: 67-9
Ondansetron 16-80mg/L in glucose 5%	Bag	Stable for 7 days at room temperature or 4°C	Eur J Cancer Clin Oncol 1989: 67-9
Ondansetron and cyclophosphamide in NaCl 0.9%	Bag (PVC)	Stable for 8 days at 4°C and 4 days at room temperature	Am J Health-Syst Pharm 1995; 52: 514-6
Ondansetron and cyclophosphamide in glucose 5%	Bag (PVC)	Stable for 8 days at 4°C and 4 days at room temperature	Am J Health-Syst Pharm 1995; 52: 514-6
Ondansetron 0.1 and 1mg/mL and hydromorphone	Glass	>31 days at 4 and 22°C and 7 days at 32°C in NaCl 0.9%	Am J Hosp Pharm 1994; 51: 2138-42
Ondansetron 0.1 and 1mg/mL and morphine 1mg/mL	Glass	>31 days at 4 and 22°C and 7 days at 32°C in NaCl 0.9%	Am J Hosp Pharm 1994; 51: 2138-42
Ondansetron 0.64mg/dexamethasone 0.2-0.4mg	Bag	In glucose 5% stable for 30 days at 4°C then 2 days at room temperature	Am J Health-Syst Pharm 1996; 53: 1431-5
Ondansetron 5-32mg/50mL in NaCl 0.9%	Bag (PVC)	Stable for 30 days at 4°C followed by 2 days at room temperature	Am J Health-Syst Pharm 1996; 53: 1431-5
Ondansetron 5-32mg/dexamethasone 10mg	Syringe	Stable for 30 days at 4°C then 2 days at room temperature	Am J Health-Syst Pharm 1996; 53: 1431-5
Ondansetron 5-32mg/dexamethasone 10-20mg	Bag (PVC)	Stable for 30 days at 4°C then 2 days at room temperature	Am J Health-Syst Pharm 1996; 53: 1431-5
Ondansetron 5-32mg/dexamethasone 20mg	Syringe	In 20 and 30mL NaCl some combinations produced a precipitate	Am J Health-Syst Pharm 1996; 53: 1431-5
Ondansetron 8-32mg, dexamethasone 20mg/in glucose 5%	Bag	Stable for 24 hours at room temperature	Am J Hosp Pharm 1993; 50: 1410-4
Ondansetron 8-32mg, dexamethasone 20mg/NaCl	Bag	Stable for 24 hours at room temperature	Am J Hosp Pharm 1993; 50: 1410-4
Ondansetron and cytarabine 30-300, 200-400mg	Bag (PVC)	Stable for >48 hours at room temperature	Am J Health-Syst Pharm 1996; 53: 1297-1300
Ondansetron and dacarbazine 0.03-0.3, 1-3mg/mL	Bag (PVC)	Stable for >48 hours at room temperature	Am J Health-Syst Pharm 1996; 53: 1297-1300
Ondansetron and doxorubicin 0.03-0.3, 1-2mg/mL	Bag (PVC)	Stable for >48 hours at room temperature	Am J Health-Syst Pharm 1996; 53: 1297-1300
Ondansetron and etoposide 30-300, 100-400mg/L	Bag (PVC)	Stable for >48 hours at room temperature	Am J Health-Syst Pharm 1996; 53: 1297-1300
Ondansetron and methotrexate 0.03-0.3, 0.5-6mg/mL	Bag (PVC)	Stable for >48 hours at room temperature	Am J Health-Syst Pharm 1996; 53: 1297-1300
Ondansetron/dexamethasone/lorazepam/in glucose 5%	Bag	Lorazepam loss >10% in 4 hours at room temperature	Am J Hosp Pharm 1993; 50: 1410-4
Ondansetron/dexamethasone/lorazepam/in NaCl 0.9%	Bag	Lorazepam loss >10% in 4 hours	Am J Hosp Pharm 1993; 50: 1410-4

Ondansetron 0.05-0.4mg/mL and cyclophosphamide 0.3-2mg/mL	Bag	Stable for 8 days at 4°C and 4 days at room temperature	Am J Health-Syst Pharm 1995; 52: 514-516
Ornidazole 1g in 100 and 250mL of NaCl 0.9%	Bag	15 days at 25°C, 30 days at 5°C	Eur J Hosp Pharm 1994; 4: 17-19
Ornidazole 1g in 100 and 250mL of glucose 5%	Bag	15 days at 25°C, 30 days at 5°C	Eur J Hosp Pharm 1994; 4: 17-19
Ornidazole 1g, gentamicin 240mg in NaCl 0.9%	Bag	30 days at 4°C and 25°C	Eur J Hosp Pharm 1994; 4: 17-19
Ornidazole 1g, gentamicin 240mg in glucose 5%	Bag	30 days at 4°C and 25°C	Eur J Hosp Pharm 1994; 4: 17-19
Oxacillin in glucose 5% or in NaCl 0.9%	Pump (PVC)	24 hours at room temperature, 7 days in fridge	Trissel
Oxytocin 10u/mL	Syringe	t95% 10 days at 4°C	Pharm J 1992; 248(Suppl): HS24-6
Paclitaxel	Admin set	Study on DEHP leaching for many administration sets	Am J Hosp Pharm 1994; 51: 2804-10
Paclitaxel 0.1 and 1mg/mL in glucose 5% and in NaCl 0.9%	Bag	Stable for 3 days at 4, 22 or 32°C precipitation may then occur	Am J Hosp Pharm 1994; 51: 3058-60
Paclitaxel 0.3 and 1.2mg/mL in glucose 5% and NaCl 0.9%	Bag (PVC)	Leached DEHP when stored for up to 8 hours at room temperature	Am J Health-Syst Pharm 1997; 54: 566-9
Paclitaxel 0.2-0.3mg/mL in glucose 5%	Bottle	Precipitation within 24 hours	Am J Hosp Pharm 1993; 50: 2518-9
Paclitaxel and ondansetron or ranitidine		4 hours in glass containers	Am J Hosp Pharm 1994; 51: 1201-4
Papaverine 12mg/mL in NaCl 0.9%	Syringe	3 months at 5°C	Hosp Pharm Pract 1992; 2: 361-2
Papaverine 1mg/mL in NaCl 0.9%	Syringe	6 months in fridge	Hosp Pharm Pract 1992; 2: 361-2
Papaverine 40mg/mL in NaCl 0.9%	Syringe	Precipitation after 1 month at 5°C	Hosp Pharm Pract 1992; 2: 361-2
Pefloxacin 1.6mg/mL 250mL in NaCl 0.9%	Bag	No significant loss at room temperature in light after 6 hours	Int J Pharmaceutics 1993; 89: 125-131
Pefloxacin 1.6mg/mL 250mL in glucose 5%	Bag	No significant loss at room temperature in light after 6 hours	Int J Pharmaceutics 1993; 89: 125-131
Penicillin G in glucose 5% or in NaCl 0.9%	Pump (PVC)	24 hours at room temperature, 7 days in fridge	Trissel
Pentamidine isethionate in NaCl 0.9%	Pump (PVC)	48 hours at room temperature, 30 days in fridge	Trissel
Pethidine 600mg/60mL in NaCl 0.9%	Syringe	No degradation after 16 days at room temperature in light	Pharm J 1992; 248(Suppl): HS24-6
Phenylephrine 0.005% in NaCl 0.9%	Syringe	No degradation after 7 days at 4°C, <5% at room temperature and 40°C	Pharm J 1992; 248(Suppl): HS24-6
Piperacillin 30mg/mL in NaCl 0.9%	Pump reservoir	No significant loss after 24 hours at 25°C and 7 days at 5°C	Am J Health-Syst Pharm 1996; 53: 2740-3
Piperacillin 30mg/mL in glucose 5%	Pump reservoir	No significant loss after 24 hours at 25°C and 4% after 7 days at 5°C	Am J Health-Syst Pharm 1996; 53: 2740-3
Piperacillin 450mg/mL in glucose 5%	Bag	30 days frozen and 7 days in fridge	Am J Hosp Pharm 1991; 48: 2184-6
Piperacillin and tazobactam infusion	Bag; syringe	See reference for details	Am J Health-Syst Pharm 1995; 52: 999
Piperacillin in glucose 5% or in NaCl 0.9%	Pump (PVC)	24 hours at room temperature, 48 hours in fridge	Trissel
Piperacillin 10g/L in NaCl 0.9%	Bag	4% loss in 48 hours, 8% in 5 days at 25°C, 2% in 28 days, 6% in 49 days at 5°C	Am J Intravenous Ther 1984: 14-19
Piperacillin 10g/L in glucose 5%	Bag	4% loss in 48 hours, 9% in 5 days at 25°C, 3% in 28 days, 8% in 49 days at 5°C	Am J Intravenous Ther 1984: 14-19
Piperacillin 2 and 3g/10mL in water	Syringe	10% loss in 2 days at 24°C and 10 days at 4°C	NITA 1987; 10: 368-72
Pirarubicin 80mg/100mL in glucose 5%	Bag	10% conversion to doxorubicin in 7 days at 4°C	Pharm Weekbl (Sci) 1992; 14: 365-9
Pirarubicin in NaCl 0.9%	Bag	Rapid precipitation	Pharm Weekbl (Sci) 1992; 14: 365-9
Procainamide 0.4 and 0.8% in glucose 5%	Bag	For 0.4% solution 6 hours at room temperature, 12 hours at 5°C; for 0.8% solution 6-12 hours at room temperature, 24 hours at 5°C	Am J Hosp Pharm 1988; 45: 2513-7
Propofol (2 piece syringe)	Syringe	2% loss in 28 days at 4°C	Pharm Pract 1997; 7: 15-6
Propofol (3 piece syringe)	Syringe	7% loss in 28 days at 4°C	Pharm Pract 1997; 7: 15-6
Propofol 2.5mg/mL in glucose 5%	Bag (PVC)	10% loss in 1 hour at room temperature and 2 days at 4°C	Int J Pharmaceutics 1996; 130: 251-5
Propofol 2.5mg/mL in glucose 5%	Bag	6% loss after 30 days at room temperature, none at 4°C	Int J Pharmaceutics 1996; 130: 251-5
Propofol and alfentanil	Syringe pump	Compatible for 6 hours	Int J Pharmaceutics 1996; 127: 255-9
Propofol and thiopental sodium 5 and 12.5mg/mL	Syringe	Stable for 13 days at 4°C and 5 days at room temperature	Am J Health-Syst Pharm 1996; 53: 1576-9
Prostaglandin injection 20µg/mL		107 days at 4°C, 9.8 days at 25°C	J Clin Pharm Ther 1995; 20: 41-44
Quinidine gluconate 300mg/50mL in glucose 5%	Bag (PVC)	40% absorption with PVC IV set	Am J Hosp Pharm 1996; 53: 655-8
Ranitidine 0.05mg/mL in glucose 10%	Bag	6.5% loss in 2 days, 11% in 7 days at room temperature	Am J Hosp Pharm 1990; 47: 1580-4
Ranitidine 0.05mg/mL in glucose 5% and NaCl 0.45%	Bag	5% loss in 2 days, 8% in 7 days at room temperature	Am J Hosp Pharm 1990; 47: 1580-4
Ranitidine 0.05mg/mL in glucose 5% and compound sodium lactate	Bag	14% loss in 2 days, 20% in 7 days at room temperature	Am J Hosp Pharm 1990; 47: 1580-4
Ranitidine 0.05mg/mL in NaCl 0.9%	Bag	2% loss in 7 days, 3% in 28 days at room temperature	Am J Hosp Pharm 1990; 47: 1580-4

Ranitidine 0.05mg/mL in glucose 5%	Bag	5% loss in 2 days, 7% in 7 days at room temperature	Am J Hosp Pharm 1990; 47: 1580-4
Ranitidine 0.5mg/mL in NaCl 0.9%	Bag	No significant loss in 28 days at room temperature	Am J Hosp Pharm 1990; 47: 1580-4
Ranitidine 0.5mg/mL in glucose 5%	Bag	2% loss in 7 days, 5% in 28 days at room temperature	Am J Hosp Pharm 1990; 47: 1580-4
Ranitidine 0.5-2mg/mL 500 mL in NaCl 0.9%	Bag	No loss in 7 days at room temperature, 30 days at 4°C, 60 days at -20°C	Am J Hosp Pharm 1990; 47: 2043-6
Ranitidine 0.5-2mg/mL in glucose 10%	Bag	3% loss in 7 days at room temperature, 2-6% after 30 days at 4°C	Am J Hosp Pharm 1990; 47: 2043-6
Ranitidine 0.5-2mg/mL in glucose 5%	Bag	5% loss in 7 days at room temperature, 2% after 30 days at 4°C	Am J Hosp Pharm 1990; 47: 2043-6
Ranitidine 0.5-2mg/mL in glucose 5%/NaCl 0.45%	Bag	3-5% loss in 7 days at room temperature, 0-8% after 30 days at 4°C	Am J Hosp Pharm 1990; 47: 2043-6
Ranitidine 0.5-2mg/mL in glucose 5%/compound sodium lactate	Bag	5% loss in 7 days at room temperature, 0-8% after 30 days at 4°C	Am J Hosp Pharm 1990; 47: 2043-6
Ranitidine 1.5mg/mL 100mL in NaCl 0.9%	Pump	> 7 days at 4°C and 24 hours at 30°C	Am J Hosp Pharm 1994; 51: 1707-8
Ranitidine 1.5mg/mL 100mL in glucose 5%	Pump	7 days at 4°C and 24 hours at 30°C	Am J Hosp Pharm 1994; 51: 1707-8
Ranitidine 1.8mg/mL in glucose 5%	Bag	2% loss in 7 days, 5% in 28 days at room temperature	Am J Hosp Pharm 1990; 47: 1580-4
Ranitidine 350mg/mL in glucose 5%	Bag	30 days frozen and 10 days in fridge	Am J Hosp Pharm 1991; 48: 2184-6
Ranitidine 50mg/mL in NaCl 0.9%	Bag	92 days at 4°C	Can J Hosp Pharm 1988; 41: 105-8
Ranitidine 50mg/mL in glucose 5%	Bag	92 days at 4°C	Can J Hosp Pharm 1988; 41: 105-8
Ranitidine 0.5-2mg/mL and aminophylline 0.5-2mg/mL in NaCl 0.9%	Bag (PVC)	Stable for 48 hours	Am J Hosp Pharm 1994; 51: 1802-7
Ranitidine 0.5-2mg/mL and dobutamine 0.25-1mg/mL in NaCl 0.9%	Bag (PVC)	Stable for 48 hours	Am J Hosp Pharm 1994; 51: 1802-7
Ranitidine 0.5-2mg/mL and dopamine 0.4-3.2mg/mL in NaCl 0.9%	Bag (PVC)	Stable for 48 hours	Am J Hosp Pharm 1994; 51: 1802-7
Ranitidine 0.5-2mg/mL and lignocaine 1-8mg/mL in NaCl 0.9%	Bag (PVC)	Stable for 48 hours	Am J Hosp Pharm 1994; 51: 1802-7
Ranitidine 0.5-2mg/mL and methylprednisolone 0.04-2mg/mL in NaCl 0.9%	Bag (PVC)	Stable for 48 hours	Am J Hosp Pharm 1994; 51: 1802-7
Ranitidine 0.5-2mg/mL and noradrenaline 0.004-0.008mg/mL in NaCl 0.9%	Bag (PVC)	Stable for 48 hours	Am J Hosp Pharm 1994; 51: 1802-7
Ranitidine 0.5-2mg/mL and sodium nitroprusside 0.05-0.4mg/mL in NaCl 0.9%	Bag (PVC)	Stable for 48 hours	Am J Hosp Pharm 1994; 51: 1802-7
Rifampicin 0.1mg/mL in NaCl 0.9%	Bag	6% loss in 3 days at 4°C, 6% at room temperature in 8 hours, 13% in 24 hours	Am J Hosp Pharm 1993; 50: 698-701
Rifampicin 0.1mg/mL in glucose 5%	Bag	8% loss in 3 days at 4°C, 5% at room temperature in 8 hours, 14% in 24 hours	Am J Hosp Pharm 1993; 50: 698-701
Rifampicin and minocycline 0.1mg/mL in glucose 5%	Bag	10% loss rifampicin in 3 days, no significant loss of minocycline in 7 days at 4°C	Am J Hosp Pharm 1993; 50: 698-701
Sodium nitroprusside and ranitidine in NaCl 0.9%	Bag (PVC)	Stable for 48 hours	Am J Hosp Pharm 1994; 51: 1802-7
Succinylcholine 20mg/mL in NaCl 0.9%	Syringe	No significant loss after 107 days at 5°C	J Clin Pharm Ther 1994; 19: 195-8
Succinylcholine 20mg/mL in glucose 5%	Syringe	No significant loss after 107 days at 5°C	J Clin Pharm Ther 1994; 19: 195-8
Sufentanil 0.5mg and bupivacaine 200mg/100mL	Pump reservoir	Bufferred NaCl (pH 4.6) no loss after 48 hours at 32°C	Pharm World Sci 1993; 15: 139-44
Sufentanil 0.5mg/100mL in NaCl 0.9%	Cassette	13% loss at 32°C in 2 days	Pharm Weekbl (Sci) 1992; 14: 196-200
Sufentanil 0.5mg/100mL in NaCl 0.9%	Bag	No significant loss in 21 days at -20, 4 and 32°C	Pharm Weekbl (Sci) 1992; 14: 196-200
Sufentanil 0.5mg/100mL in NaCl 0.9%	Cassette	Precipitate at 4°C but no degradation after 21 days	Pharm Weekbl (Sci) 1992; 14: 196-200
Sufentanil 0.5mg/100mL in NaCl 0.9%	Glass	<5% loss in 21 days at -20, 4 and 32°C	Pharm Weekbl (Sci) 1992; 14: 196-200
Sufentanil 0.5mg/100mL in NaCl 0.9% with citrate buffer (pH4)	Pump reservoir	5% loss due to absorption after 21 days at 32°C	Pharm World Sci 1993; 15: 139-44
Sufentanil 0.5mg/100mL in NaCl 0.9% with citrate buffer (pH5)	Pump reservoir	24% loss due to absorption after 21 days at 32	Pharm World Sci 1993; 15: 139-44
Sufentanil 0.5mg/100mL in NaCl 0.9%	Pump reservoir	11% loss due to absorption in 48 hours at 32°C	Pharm World Sci 1993; 15: 139-44
Sufentanil 5µg/mL in glucose 5%	Pump	Stable for 30 days at 5°C and 3 days at 32°C	Pharm World Sci 1993; 15: 269-75
Sufentanil 0.5mg/100mL in NaCl 0.9% with citrate buffer (pH4.6)	Pump reservoir	5% loss due to absorption after 21 days at 32°C	Pharm World Sci 1993; 15: 139-44
Sufentanil 0.5mg/100mL in NaCl 0.9% with citrate buffer (pH5.6)	Pump reservoir	52% loss due to absorption after 21days at 32	Pharm World Sci 1993; 15: 139-44
Sufentanil 5µg/mL and bupivacaine 2mg/mL in NaCl 0.9%	Pump	Stable for 30 days at 5°C and 3 days at 32°C	Pharm World Sci 1993; 15: 269-75
Sufentanil 20µg/mL in 0.3% bupivacaine	Cassette	No significant loss after 10 days at 26°C	Eur Hosp Pharm 1995; 1: 12-14

Sufentanil 20µg/mL in NaCl 0.9%	Cassette	10% loss in 2 days at 26°C, 18% at 37°C	Eur Hosp Pharm 1995; 1: 12-14
Sulbactam 10mg/ampicillin 20mg/mL in NaCl 0.9%	Bag	10% loss in ampicillin in 60 hours at 5°C, 24 hours at 24°C	Am J Hosp Pharm 1994; 51: 901-4
Sulbactam/ampicillin/aztreonam/in NaCl 0.9%	Bag	10% loss in ampicillin in 84 hours at 5°C, 30 hours at 24°C	Am J Hosp Pharm 1994; 51: 901-4
Tacrolimus 10µg and cimetidine 600µg/mL in NaCl 0.9%		Stable for 48 hours at 22-26°C	Am J Health-Syst Pharm 1995; 52: 2024-5
Tacrolimus 10µg/mL in NaCl 0.9%		Stable for 48 hours at 22-26°C	Am J Health-Syst Pharm 1995; 52: 2024-5
Tauromustine in NaCl	Bag	Half-life of 105.9 hours at room temperature	Int J Pharmaceutics 1989; 56: 37-41
Teicoplanin 25mg/L in dialysis solution	Bag	Stable for 42 days at 4°C, 25 days at 25°C and 7 days at 37°C	Int J Pharm Pract 1993; 1: 90-3
Teicoplanin 25mg/L in dialysis solution	Bag	Stable for 7 days at 4°C then 16 hours at 25°C and 8 hours at 37	Am J Health-Syst Pharm 1996; 53: 2731-4
Teicoplanin 60mg and ciprofloxacin 2mg/mL	Y-site	Incompatible	Ann Pharmacother 1993; 27: 704-7
Teicoplanin, ceftazidime 25, 100mg/L dialysis solution	Bag	Unstable at 25°C	Am J Health-Syst Pharm 1996; 53: 2731-4
Teniposide 400mg/L in NaCl 0.9%	Bag	2-4% loss in 4 days in light at 21°C	J Parenter Sci Technol 1991; 45: 108-12
Teniposide 400mg/L in glucose 5%	Bag	6% loss in 4 days in light at 21°C	J Parenter Sci Technol 1991; 45: 108-12
Terbutaline 1mg/mL	Syringe	5-6% loss in 60 days at 4°C and room temperature in dark	Am J Hosp Pharm 1987; 44: 2291-3
Terbutaline 30mg/L in NaCl 0.9%	Bag	<10% loss at room temperature in light	Am J Hosp Pharm 1986; 43: 1760-2
Terbutaline 30mg/L in glucose 5%	Bag	<10% loss at room temperature in light	Am J Hosp Pharm 1986; 43: 1760-2
Tetracycline in glucose 5% or in NaCl 0.9%	Pump (PVC)	12 hours at room temperature	Trissel
Thiopental sodium and propofol 12.5 and 5mg/mL	Syringe	Stable for 13 days at 4°C and 5 days at room temperature	Am J Health-Syst Pharm 1996; 53: 1576-9
Thiopentone sodium 500mg/20mL in water	Syringe	21 days in fridge	Pharm J 1992; 248(Suppl): HS20-1
Thiotepa 0.5mg/mL in glucose 5%	Bag (PVC)	<5% loss at 4°C and <7% at 23°C after 8 hours, 12% at 24 hours	Am J Health-Syst Pharm 1996; 53: 2728-30
Thiotepa 0.5mg/mL in glucose 5%	Bag	10% loss after 8 hours at 4 and 23°C, 15% at 24 hours	Am J Health-Syst Pharm 1996; 53: 2728-30
Thiotepa 5mg/mL in glucose 5%	Bag	10% loss after 14 days at 4°C and 3 days at 23°C	Am J Health-Syst Pharm 1996; 53: 2728-30
Thiotepa 5mg/mL in glucose 5%	Bag (PVC)	10% loss after 14 days at 4°C and 3 days at 23°C	Am J Health-Syst Pharm 1996; 53: 2728-30
Ticarcillin 25, 100mg/mL, in NaCl 0.45% and in water	Syringe	No significant loss after 7 days at 4°C, 30 days at -20°C, 24 hours at room temperature	Am J Health-Syst Pharm 1995; 52: 890-2
Ticarcillin and clavulanate in glucose 5% or NaCl 0.9%	Pump (PVC)	24 hours at room temperature, 7 days in fridge	Trissel
Tobramycin 0.8mg/mL in NaCl 0.9%	Pump reservoir	No significant loss after 24 hours at 25°C	Am J Health-Syst Pharm 1996; 53: 2740-3
Tobramycin 120mg in glucose 5% and in NaCl 0.9%	Bag	Stable for 48 hours at room temperature and 4°C	Am J Hosp Pharm 1991; 48: 2166-71
Tobramycin 40mg/mL	Syringe	No significant loss after 2 months at room temperature and 4°C	Am J Hosp Pharm 1980; 37: 1614
Tobramycin 60 and 120mg/20mL in glucose 10%	Vial	No significant degradation after 30 days	Am J Hosp Pharm 1994; 51: 518-9
Tobramycin in glucose 5% or in NaCl 0.9%	Pump (PVC)	48 hours at room temperature, 96 hours in fridge	Trissel
Tobramycin and ciprofloxacin 120/200mg/100mL NaCl 0.9%	Bag	Both stable for 24 hours at room temperature and 4°C	Am J Hosp Pharm 1991; 48: 2166-71
Tobramycin and ciprofloxacin 120/200mg/100mL glucose 5%	Bag	Both stable for 24 hours at room temperature and 4°C	Am J Hosp Pharm 1991; 48: 2166-71
Tolazoline 8mg and dopamine 1mg/mL in glucose 10%	Infusion	<5% degradation for dopamine, no degradation for tolazoline in 24 hours at room temperature	Hosp Pharm Pract 1992; 3: 205-210
Tolazoline 8mg and dopamine 1mg/mL	Infusion	<7% degradation for dopamine, no degradation for tolazoline in 24 hours at room temperature	Hosp Pharm Pract 1992; 3: 205-210
Vancomycin 1000mg/250mL in glucose 5%	Bag	9% loss in 30 days at 4°C, 8% in 17 days at room temperature	Can J Hosp Pharm 1988; 41: 233-8
Vancomycin 1000mg/250mL in NaCl 0.9%	Bag	5% loss in 30 days at 4°C, 10% in 24 days at room temperature	Can J Hosp Pharm 1988; 41: 233-8
Vancomycin 10mg and aztreonam 40mg/mL	Bag (PVC)	Incompatible in glucose 5% and in NaCl 0.9%	Am J Hosp Pharm 1995; 52: 2560-4
Vancomycin 10mg/mL in water	Pump reservoir	24 hours at 5°C and 30°C	Am J Hosp Pharm 1995; 52: 70-4
Vancomycin 10mg/mL in water	Pump reservoir	24 hours at 5°C and 30°C	Am J Hosp Pharm 1995; 52: 70-4
Vancomycin 1mg and aztreonam 4mg/mL in NaCl 0.9%	Bag (PVC)	31 days at 4°C and 23°C and 7 days at 32°C	Am J Hosp Pharm 1995; 52: 2560-4
Vancomycin 1mg and aztreonam 4mg/mL in glucose 5%	Bag (PVC)	31 days at 4°C, 14 days at 23°C and 7 days at 32°C	Am J Hosp Pharm 1995; 52: 2560-4
Vancomycin 25 and 50mg and cefotaxime 100mg/mL	Y-site	Incompatible	Am J Hosp Pharm 1993; 50: 2057-8

Vancomycin 500mg/100mL in NaCl 0.9%	Bag	5% loss in 30 days at 4°C, 8.5% in 24 days at room temperature	Can J Hosp Pharm1988; 41: 233-8
Vancomycin 500mg/100mL in glucose 5%	Bag	9% loss in 30 days at 4°C, 8% in 17 days at room temperature	Can J Hosp Pharm1988; 41: 233-8
Vancomycin 5mg/mL in NaCl 0.9%	Bag (PVC)	No significant loss after 7 days at 4°C or 48 hours at 22°C	Int J Pharmaceutics 1996; 139: 243-7
Vancomycin 5mg/mL in glucose 5%.	Bag (PVC)	No significant loss after 7 days at 4°C or 48 hours at 22°C	Int J Pharmaceutics 1996; 139: 243-7
Vancomycin 5mg/mL in NaCl 0.9%	Pump reservoir	No significant loss after 24 hours at 25°C and 14 days at 5°C	Am J Health-Syst Pharm 1996; 53: 2740-3
Vancomycin 5mg/mL in glucose 5%	Pump reservoir	2% loss after 24 hours at 25°C and 3% after 14 days at 5°C	Am J Health-Syst Pharm 1996; 53: 2740-3
Vancomycin in glucose 5% or in NaCl 0.9%	Pump (PVC)	7 days at room temperature, 2 weeks in fridge	Trissel
Vinblastine 10mg/250mL in NaCl 0.9%	Bag	Stable for 7 days at 4°C	Int J Pharmaceutics 1991; 77: 279-285
Vinblastine 10mg/250mL in glucose 5%	Bag	Stable for 7 days at 4°C	Int J Pharmaceutics 1991; 77: 279-285
Vincristine 2mg/250mL in NaCl 0.9%	Bag	Stable for 7 days at 4°C	Int J Pharmaceutics 1991; 77: 279-285
Vincristine 2mg/250mL in glucose 5%	Bag	Stable for 7 days at 4°C	Int J Pharmaceutics 1991; 77: 279-285
Vincristine1.6mg and mitozantrone 16mg in NaCl 0.9%	Cassette	4 days at room temperature	Pharm J 1992; 248(Suppl): HS40-1
Vindesine 4mg/250mL in NaCl 0.9%	Bag	Stable for 7 days at 4°C	Int J Pharmaceutics 1991; 77: 279-285
Vindesine 4mg/250mL in glucose 5%	Bag	Stable for 7 days at 4°C	Int J Pharmaceutics 1991; 77: 279-285
Vinorelbine 50mg/250mL in NaCl 0.9%	Bag	Stable for 3 days at 4°C	Int J Pharmaceutics 1991; 77: 279-285
Vinorelbine 50mg/250mL in glucose 5%	Bag	Stable for 7 days at 4°C	Int J Pharmaceutics 1991; 77: 279-285
Warfarin sodium 2.5mg/100mL in NaCl 0.9%	Bag	No significant loss after 120 hours at room temperature	Int J Pharmaceutics 1994; 110: 197-201
Warfarin sodium 2.5mg/100mL in NaCl 0.9%	Bag (PVC)	50% loss in 20 hours at pH 4.9 and 20% at pH 5.6 at room temperature	Int J Pharmaceutics 1994; 110: 197-201
Zidovudine 4mg/mL in NaCl 0.9%	Bag	98% remaining after 8 days at room temperature and in fridge	Am J Hosp Pharm 1991; 48: 280-2
Zidovudine 4mg/mL in glucose 5%	Bag	98% remaining after 8 days at room temperature and in fridge	Am J Hosp Pharm 1991; 48: 280-2
Zorubicin 1mg/mL in NaCl 0.9%	Bag	10% degradation to daunorubicin at 4°C in 6 hours	J Pharm Biomed Anal 1996; 14: 695-705
Zorubicin 1mg/mL in glucose 5%	Bag	10% degradation to daunorubicin at 4°C in 4 hours	J Pharm Biomed Anal 1996; 14: 695-705
Zorubicin 250µg/mL in glucose 5% or NaCl 0.9%	Bag	>10% degradation in <15 minutes at 4°C	J Pharm Biomed Anal 1996; 14: 695-705

Note:
1. ABPI. Data sheet 1996-97 is 'ABPI. Compendium of data sheets and summaries of product characteristics 1996-97. London: Datapharm Publications Ltd, 1996.'
2. Trissel is 'Trissel LA, editor. Handbook on injectable drugs, 7th edition. Bethesda, MD: American Society of Hospital Pharmacists, 1992.'

8 CIVAS Drug Monographs

Tim Sizer

8.1 Introduction

It has long been recognised that there are problems associated with the safe and effective administration of intravenous drugs. This is discussed elsewhere in the *Handbook*, and the principal issues involved were fully and clearly expressed in the report of the working party on the addition of drugs to intravenous infusion fluids chaired by Professor Breckenridge in 1976.

Ideally, all intravenous drug preparations would be available in a ready-to-use form, but this is never likely to be achieved. Stability, packaging, concentration and volume, drug combinations, and variations in diluents, are all issues that limit the ability of the commercial supplier to provide ready to use drug presentations. There is, and will continue to be, a need for the bespoke preparation of intravenous drugs, whether at the patients bedside or in a centralised facility.

Intravenous drug therapy is not a simple matter and involves many complex issues. With an ever increasing range of active drug substances and a variety of presentations available, it can be difficult to correctly select and prescribe the appropriate route, mode, and duration of administration. The process is further complicated by the choice of diluent and the assignment of a shelf-life for an admixture. These decisions can be particularly difficult when there is a need or a desire to administer a drug by a method, or in a concentration or solution, that is outside the recommendations provided by the manufacturers data sheet or summary of product characteristics. A situation which, to those involved in the provision of CIVAS, seems to occur with increasing frequency.

Usually, it is the role of hospital pharmacy departments to provide suitable solutions to drug administration problems. However, information on which to base a decision is often difficult to find or interpret. Such data that is available must often be considered with great care and even then, pharmacists and prescribers may have to rely on an 'educated guess' and trust that what they decide will not cause undue harm to the patient.

The potency and complexity of many drug formulations now in use increases the risk of problems, particularly in the processes of reconstitution and administration. Decisions on the safety and stability of any particular intravenous drug admixture are correspondingly more difficult to make and it is therefore vital that those concerned have a sound understanding of the factors involved in the formulation, stability, and degradation of these products. This is discussed elsewhere, but one of the main objectives of this *Handbook* is to assist in the decision making process, and the monographs in this section have been compiled as an aid to producing the required therapy in a form that is both safe and effective.

The list of drugs for which monographs have been prepared is far from complete, but those that have been included represent an attempt to meet the information needs expressed by pharmacists currently working in CIVAS. It is anticipated that further monographs will be added in subsequent editions, and contributions and comments are actively welcomed by the editors.

Many authors have participated in the *Handbook* project, and every attempt has been made to collate high quality information, and to verify accuracy. In addition, each of the monographs has been the subject of peer review. Nevertheless, the body of scientific knowledge drawn upon to draft these texts is constantly being updated and extended, and the use and interpretation of the information given is more subjective than objective, dependent upon individual circumstances.

In general, the usage and stability information quoted or summarised in the monographs are applicable only if the product or admixture has been prepared in a manner similar to that described, in the carefully monitored and controlled conditions of an aseptic facility, by suitably trained operators.

Readers are assumed to possess the necessary knowledge to interpret the information contained within the *Handbook* and are encouraged to check original sources for themselves and to consider local circumstances carefully before applying the information. The authors, editors, and publisher, cannot accept any responsibility for the interpretation of the monographs by others.

8.2 List of Drug Monographs

Aciclovir

Approved Name
Aciclovir

UK Proprietary Name
Zovirax (Glaxo Wellcome)

Other Names
Acyclovir.

Product Details
Glass vials containing the equivalent of 250 mg and 500 mg of aciclovir as the freeze-dried sodium salt. Sodium content is 1 mmol per 250 mg. The pH of the reconstituted product is 11.[1] Displacement volume is negligible.

Preparation of Injection
The contents of the vial are reconstituted by dissolving in sodium chloride 0.9% or water for injection, 10 mL for the 250 mg vial or 20 mL for the 500 mg vial, to provide a solution containing aciclovir 25 mg/mL. The required volume of reconstituted solution may then be further diluted to give an aciclovir concentration of not greater than 5 mg/mL. Suitable infusion fluids are: compound sodium lactate; sodium chloride 0.45%; sodium chloride 0.9%; sodium chloride 0.18% and glucose 4%; and sodium chloride 0.45% and glucose 2.5%.

Solutions should be discarded if any turbidity or crystallisation is observed.[1]

Administration
Aciclovir should be administered by intravenous infusion over a one-hour period.

Stability in Practice
The reconstituted injection containing aciclovir 25 mg/mL, or the injection after dilution in the recommended infusions, is stable at 20°C for up to 12 hours.[1] Refrigeration of the reconstituted solution or diluted infusion is not recommended because precipitation may occur.[1]

Reconstituted aciclovir is relatively stable in strongly alkaline solutions. Stability and physical compatibility of aciclovir after reconstitution is dependent on drug concentration and temperature.

Published Information The chemical stability of aciclovir 5 mg/mL in glucose 5% and sodium chloride 0.9% stored in PVC infusion bags was investigated.[2] Analysis was by HPLC assay. Samples were stored at 5°C for up to 37 days. Results indicated no detectable loss of aciclovir at 5°C or at 25°C after 37 days storage in PVC bags. The pH range of the solutions fell from 10–10.6 to 9.7–10.2. There was no visible evidence of precipitation during the study at 5°C or 25°C.

The stability of aciclovir was investigated in sodium chloride 0.9% in PVC minibags and in EVA bags at concentrations of 500 mg/100 mL and 250 mg/100 mL at 25°C. The results showed that there was no significant decomposition over 28 days at 25°C. However, a significant increase in particle load was recorded for aciclovir stored in the PVC bags, this was apparently due to an interaction between the high pH infusion fluid and the PVC bag. There was no such increase for infusions stored in EVA bags.[3]

Unpublished Information The chemical stability of aciclovir in sodium chloride 0.9% stored in 10 mL plastic syringes containing aciclovir 25 mg/mL and in 100 mL PVC minibags containing aciclovir 5 mg/mL was investigated. Analysis was by stability indicating HPLC assay. Storage was at refrigeration temperature (not specified) and 23°C for up to five days for the syringes and 28 days for the minibags, in the dark. Results indicated that solutions stored in polypropylene syringes appeared to degrade when stored at 23°C, the $t_{90\%}$ value quoted being 4.4 days, while solutions stored at refrigeration temperatures showed evidence of precipitation within two days. Solutions stored in minibags showed no evidence of degradation after 28 days storage at refrigeration temperature or 23°C and retained physical compatibility.[4]

The addition of glucose 5% to reconstituted aciclovir injection results in an increase in particle count within eight hours and a reduction in pH, thereby increasing the risk of precipitation.[5]

Aciclovir sodium 10 mg/mL in sodium chloride 0.9% was reported to be stable for 10 days, at room temperature, 30 days refrigerated in an elastomeric infusion system. However, the drugs potential for precipitation at low temperature and in certain conditions and pH was noted.[6]

Incompatibilities Aciclovir sodium solutions have been shown to be physically or chemically incompatible with the following drug substances: amsacrine; cefepime hydrochloride; diltiazem hydrochloride; dobutamine hydrochloride; dopamine hydrochloride; fludarabine phosphate; foscarnet sodium; idarubicin hydrochloride; morphine sulphate; ondansetron hydrochloride; pethidine hydrochloride; piperacillin-tazobactam sodium; sargramostim; and vinorelbine tartrate.[7] Aciclovir is also stated to be incompatible with solutions containing hydroxybenzoates.

Compatibilities Specialist references should be consulted for specific compatibility data.[7]

Comments

Information currently available suggests that solutions containing aciclovir 25 mg/mL in plastic syringes should be used within 12 hours of preparation and should not be refrigerated.[5] Solutions diluted in sodium chloride 0.9% PVC minibags to a concentration of 5 mg/mL may be stored for 28 days at room temperature, protected from light, but storage will result in a significant increase in the particle load of the product.[3]

Infusions containing other concentrations of aciclovir should not be stored for more than 12 hours unless further data is available.

References

1. ABPI. Compendium of data sheets and summaries of product characteristics 1996-1997. London: Datapharm Publications Ltd, 1996: 1219-20.
2. Das Gupta V, Pramar Y, Bethea C. Stability of acyclovir sodium in dextrose and sodium chloride injections. J Clin Pharm Ther 1989; 14: 451-6.
3. McLaughlin JP, Simpson C, Taylor RA. How stable is acyclovir in PVC minibags? Pharm in Pract 1995; 5(2): 53-9.
4. Frary A, Adams P. Personal communication, 1997.
5. Glaxo Wellcome Ltd. Personal communication, 1996.
6. Block Medical Inc. Personal communication, 1996.
7. Trissel LA. Handbook on injectable drugs, 9th edition. Bethesda, MD: American Society of Health-System Pharmacists Inc, 1996: 5-8.

Prepared by

Charlotte Gibb

Alfentanil

Approved Name

Alfentanil hydrochloride

UK Proprietary Name

Rapifen (Janssen-Cilag Ltd)
Rapifen Intensive Care (Janssen-Cilag Ltd)

Other Names

—

Product Details

Aqueous injections of 2 mL and 10 mL which are preservative free, clear and colourless and contain 500 μg/mL of alfentanil as the hydrochloride. The 1 mL injection (Rapifen Intensive Care) contains alfentanil 5 mg/mL as the hydrochloride. Both strengths contain 0.15 mmol/mL of sodium.[1] Store at room temperature; pH from 4–6;[2] shelf-life five years.[1] Alfentanil is a controlled drug.

Preparation of Injection

The ampoules contain a ready-to-use intravenous injection. The 500 μg/mL solution may be used undiluted or infused with glucose 5% or sodium chloride 0.9%. The 5 mg/mL injection should be diluted with sodium chloride 0.9% before use.

Administration

In non-ventilated patients, alfentanil is given as an intravenous bolus dose over 30 seconds (dilution may be helpful). In ventilated patients, it may be given as a bolus followed by intravenous increments or infusion, or as an intravenous infusion throughout.[3]

Stability in Practice

Alfentanil is a synthetic derivative of fentanyl and is a tertiary amine. It has an ionisation constant of 6.5, resulting in approximately 10% ionisation at physiological pH.[4]

Alfentanil hydrochloride 25 mg in 50 mL of glucose 5% remains chemically stable in plastic syringes at room temperature and 8°C for at least three months.

The presence of light has no significant effect on the stability of alfentanil and the solution remains clear and colourless during storage.[5]

Published Information The stability of alfentanil hydrochloride diluted in glucose 5% has been investigated using HPLC. A variety of intravenous solutions containing alfentanil 0.5 mg/mL were stored at 8°C and room temperature (20°C) for 16 weeks. An assessment of alfentanil degradation, pH, and leaching showed that alfentanil hydrochloride 0.5 mg/mL was stable at 8°C and room temperature for at least three months.[5]

Incompatibilities Alfentanil hydrochloride has been reported to be incompatible with the following drug substances: methohexitone sodium;[1] and thiopentone sodium.[2]

Compatibilities Specialist references should be consulted for specific compatibility information.[2] Alfentanil hydrochloride is physically and chemically compatible with the following intravenous solutions: compound sodium lactate; glucose 5%; and sodium chloride 0.9%.[2,3]

Alfentanil hydrochloride has been reported to be compatible with the following drug substances: atracurium besylate;[2] bupivacaine hydrochloride;[6] droperidol;[7] etomidate;[2] midazolam;[8,9] pancuronium bromide;[1] propofol;[10,11] and suxamethonium chloride.[1]

Comments

Alfentanil hydrochloride injection is stable at room temperature. It is also stable in plastic bags after dilution to 10 μg/mL in sodium chloride 0.9%. Compatibility with some other drugs has been investigated; reported results should be interpreted with caution.

References

1. Janssen-Cilag Ltd. Personal communication, 1996.
2. Trissel LA. Handbook on injectable drugs, 9th edition. Bethesda, MD: American Society of Health-System Pharmacists Inc, 1996: 12.
3. ABPI. Compendium of data sheets and summaries of product characteristics 1996-1997. London: Datapharm Publications Ltd, 1996: 465-7.
4. Larijani GE, Goldberg ME. Alfentanil hydrochloride: a new short-acting narcotic analgesic for surgical procedures. Clin Pharm 1987; 6: 275-82.

5. Mehta AC, Petty DR, Kay EA. How stable is alfentanil: stability of alfentanil hydrochloride in 5% dextrose stored in syringes. Pharm in Pract 1995; 5(7): 303-4.

6. Cooper RA, et al. Epidural analgesia for labour using a continuous infusion of bupivacaine and alfentanil. Eur J Anaesthesiol 1993; 10: 183-7.

7. Coley S, et al. A comparison of the effects of alfentanil/droperidol on intra-ocular pressure. Anaesthesia 1990; 45: 477-80.

8. Hopkinson RB, O'Dea J. The combination alfentanil-midazolam by infusion: use for sedation in intensive therapy. Eur J Anaesthesiol 1987; 4(Suppl 1): 67-70.

9. O'Dea J, Hopkinson RB. Alfentanil-midazolam infusion. Care Crit Ill 1987; 3(1): 20-1.

10. Goodman NW, Vanner RG, Wade JA. Effects of incremental doses of alfentanil and propofol on the breathing of anaesthetized patients. Br J Anaesth 1989; 63: 548-53.

11. Sherry E. Admixture of propofol and alfentanil. Anaesthesia 1992; 47: 477-9.

Prepared by

Amanda Carthew

Amikacin

Approved Name
Amikacin

UK Proprietary Name
Amikin (Bristol-Myers Squibb)

Other Names
—

Product Details
Glass vials containing amikacin 500mg/2mL and 100mg/2mL as the sulphate. Sodium content is less than 0.5mmol/vial. The injection has a pH of 3.5–5.5. Excipients include sodium bisulphite, sodium citrate, sulphuric acid, and water. The product contains no preservative.[1]

Preparation of Injection
The vials contain a ready-to-use solution for intramuscular or slow intravenous injection. If an infusion is required, the injection may be further diluted using: compound sodium lactate; compound sodium lactate with glucose 5%; glucose 5%; or sodium chloride 0.9%. Infusions should be administered over 30 minutes (e.g. 0.25%, 250mg in 100mL).[1]

Administration
See above.

Stability in Practice
The manufacturer states that any diluted product should be used as soon as possible and not stored.[1]
Published Information It has been reported that aqueous solutions of amikacin 37.5–250mg/mL retained 90% potency for up to 36 months at 25°C.[2] Amikacin was found to be stable at concentrations of 0.025% and 0.5% in a variety of fluids including glucose 5% and sodium chloride 0.9% when stored at: 4°C for 60 days, then 25°C for 24 hours; frozen at -15°C for 30 days, thawed, then stored at 25°C for 24 hours; and frozen at -15°C for 30 days, thawed, then stored at 4°C for 24 hours, then at 25°C for 24 hours.[3]

Aqueous solutions of amikacin sulphate may darken in colour due to oxidation, but this is stated to have no effect on potency.[2]

Amikacin 750mg diluted with sodium chloride 0.9% to a final volume of 4mL was stable, showing a 2% loss of amikacin when stored in polypropylene syringes for 48 hours at 25°C under fluorescent light.[4] Amikacin 1g/50mL subjected to room temperature or microwave radiation exhibited no evidence of precipitation and showed no more than 6% potency loss (determined microbiologically). Subsequent storage at room temperature for 24 hours led to no additional loss of activity.[5]

Amikacin 250mg/21mL and 500mg/22mL solutions in glucose 10%, stored in glass vials, were found to be stable for 30 days when refrigerated.[6]
Unpublished Information Amikacin sodium 10mg/mL in sodium chloride 0.9% was reported to be stable in an elastomeric infusion device for 24 hours at room temperature, ten days refrigerated, or 30 days when frozen.[7]
Incompatibilities Amikacin has been reported to be physically or chemically incompatible with the following drug substances: allopurinol; amphotericin B; ampicillin; chlorothiazide; heparin; phenytoin; thiopentone sodium; and Pabrinex.
Compatibilities Specialist references should be consulted for specific compatibility information.[8]

The physical compatibility of amikacin 2mg/mL with frusemide 0.16mg in a PVC minibag has been reported. However, cloudiness was briefly observed at the point of injection of the frusemide into the solution.[9]

Comments
Studies indicate amikacin to be stable for up to 60 days at 4°C, and 30 days when frozen, at a range of concentrations in PVC bags. Limited information on dilution in syringes indicates 48 hours stability. In the US, pre-filled syringes of 250mg/mL are commercially available.[8]

References
1. ABPI. Compendium of data sheets and summaries of product characteristics 1996-1997. London: Datapharm Publications Ltd, 1996: 167-8.
2. Kaplan MA, et al. Pharmaceutical properties and stability of amikacin: part I. Curr Ther Res 1976; 20: 352-8.

3. Nunning BC, Granatek AP. Physical compatibility and chemical stability of amikacin sulfate in large volume parenteral solutions. Curr Ther Res 1976; 20: 359-68.

4. Zbrozek AS, et al. Compatibility and stability of clindamycin phosphate-aminoglycoside combinations within polypropylene syringes. Drug Intell Clin Pharm 1987; 21: 806-10.

5. Holmes CJ, et al. Effect of freezing and microwave thawing on the stability of six antibiotic admixtures in plastic bags. Am J Hosp Pharm 1982; 39: 104-8.

6. Wolff DJ, Kline SS, Mauro LS. Stability of amikacin, gentamicin or tobramycin in 10% dextrose injection. Am J Hosp Pharm 1994; 51: 518-9.

7. Block Medical Inc. Personal communication, 1996.

8. Trissel LA. Handbook on injectable drugs, 9th edition. Bethesda, MD: American Society of Health-System Pharmacists Inc, 1996: 14-24.

9. Thompson DF, et al. Compatibility of furosemide with aminoglycoside admixtures. Am J Hosp Pharm 1985; 42: 116-9.

Prepared by

Christine Clarke

Aminophylline

Approved Name
Aminophylline

UK Proprietary Name
None (Suppliers: Antigen; Evans; Phoenix; Martindale.)

Other Names
Theophylline and ethylenediamine.

Note: aminophylline is a stable 2:1 complex of theophylline and ethylenediamine; the ethylenediamine confers greater solubility in water. Aminophylline 25 mg is equivalent to 19.7–21.85 mg of theophylline.[1,2]

Product Details
Snap-break ampoules containing aminophylline in water for injection in the following strengths: 2 mg/mL; 5 mg/5 mL; 10 mg/mL; 10 mg/2 mL; 10 mg/5 mL; 20 mg/mL; 50 mg/5 mL; 250 mg/10 mL; and 500 mg/2 mL.

The injection has a pH of 8.8–10.0, and is sodium free.

The osmolality of a 2.5 mg/mL solution in sodium chloride 0.9% is 318 mosmol/kg, and 291 mosmol/kg in glucose 5%.[3]

Preparation of Injection
—

Administration
By slow intravenous injection over 20–30 minutes. Acute toxicity (seizures, coma, cardiac standstill, ventricular fibrillation, death) is caused by rapidity of injection rather than dose.

For prolonged intravenous infusion, injections should be diluted with compound sodium lactate, glucose 5%, or sodium chloride 0.9%. Solutions are stable for 24 hours at room temperature in water for injection or glucose 5–20% at 250 µg/mL concentration, and in glucose 5% or sodium chloride 0.9% at 1 mg/mL concentration.

Aminophylline may also be administered by deep intramuscular injection (500 mg/2 mL), although this is not suitable for children.

Stability in Practice
Injections should be protected from light and stored at a temperature less than 30°C. Refrigerated storage is not recommended due to possible reduction in solubility with crystallisation.[4] Upon exposure to air, aminophylline solutions gradually lose ethylenediamine, absorb carbon dioxide, and liberate free theophylline.[5] Containers should be inspected for particulate matter and discoloration prior to use and should not be used if crystals are present.

With glucose injection, a yellow colour may develop after two hours at room temperature. This is postulated to be due to a reaction between glucose and ethylenediamine. However, theophylline content does not decrease significantly unless the solution becomes very yellow in colour.[6]

For aminophylline 0.45 mg/mL in glucose 5%, stability is reported to be maintained over the pH range 3.5–8.6 for up to 48 hours at 25°C,[5,7] although it has also been reported that theophylline crystals may deposit below pH 8.[8]

No loss due to sorption onto PVC bags, PVC tubing, infusion sets, polyethylene tubing, silastic tubing, polypropylene syringes, or polypropylene/polystyrene syringes has been found to occur.[2,9]

The commercial products have a shelf-life of 24–36 months.

Published Information Aminophylline 5 mg/mL in water for injection stored in plastic syringes at 22°C and 4°C was stable for at least 91 days.[10] Aminophylline was stable for at least 24 hours under fluorescent lighting at room temperature in: glucose 5%; glucose 5% or glucose 20% in 50 mL polypropylene syringes, or glass flasks at 250 µg/mL concentration;[11] glucose 4% and sodium chloride 0.18%, or sodium chloride 0.9% injection, in 250 mL bags at 1 mg/mL concentration;[6] TPN solutions in minibags at 29.3 µg/mL concentration;[11] and water for injection.

Unpublished Information Aminophylline infusion 5 mg/mL and 12.5 mg/mL in sodium chloride 0.9% stored in CADD-Plus cassettes was stable for up to seven days at 37°C, and 14 days at 4°C.

Incompatibilities Aminophylline is incompatible

with the following drug substances: adrenaline hydrochloride; ascorbic acid; amiodarone hydrochloride; benzylpenicillin potassium; bleomycin sulphate; cefapirin sodium; cephalothin sodium; cephalothin sodium plus hydrocortisone sodium succinate; chlorpromazine hydrochloride; ciprofloxacin; clarithromycin;[12] clindamycin phosphate; codeine phosphate; corticotrophin; dimenhydrinate; dobutamine hydrochloride; doxapram hydrochloride; doxorubicin; erythromycin gluceptate; hydralazine hydrochloride; hydroxyzine hydrochloride; insulin (regular); isoprenaline hydrochloride; levorphanol tartrate; methadone hydrochloride; morphine sulphate; noradrenaline acid tartrate; oxytetracycline hydrochloride; papaverine hydrochloride plus trimecaine hydrochloride; pentazocine lactate; pethidine hydrochloride; procaine hydrochloride; phenytoin sodium; prochlorperazine salts; promazine hydrochloride; promethazine hydrochloride; sulphafurazole diethanolamine; tetracycline; vancomycin hydrochloride; verapamil hydrochloride; and vitamin B complex with vitamin C.

With lactose, a yellow or brown colour develops on standing; in the presence of copper, solutions develop a blue colour.

Compatibilities Ranitidine hydrochloride 0.05 mg/mL or 2 mg/mL plus aminophylline 0.5 mg/mL or 2 mg/mL were found to be stable for at least 48 hours at 25°C, both in glucose 5% and sodium chloride 0.9%.[13]

Cefuroxime sodium 7.5 mg/mL or 15.0 mg/mL and aminophylline 1 mg/mL or 2 mg/mL were stable in glucose 5%, glucose 5% and sodium chloride 0.9%, glucose 5% and sodium chloride 0.45%, and sodium chloride 0.9%, in glass bottles at 22°C for up to four hours.[14]

Fluconazole 0.5 mg/mL or 1.5 mg/mL and aminophylline 1 mg/mL or 2 mg/mL in glucose 5% or sodium chloride 0.9% were stable for at least three hours at 24°C.[15]

Cimetidine hydrochloride 1.2 mg/mL and aminophylline 0.5 mg/mL were stable in glucose 5% for 48 hours at 25°C.[16]

Methylprednisolone sodium succinate 2 mg/mL and aminophylline 1 mg/mL were stable in glucose 5% and sodium chloride 0.9%, in glass, for three hours and two hours at 25°C, respectively. Methylprednisolone sodium succinate 0.5 mg/mL and aminophylline 1 mg/mL were stable for three hours in glucose 5% and one hour in sodium chloride 0.9%.[17]

Comments

Aminophylline infusion is stable for 24 hours at 25°C in glucose 5–20%, glucose 4% and sodium chloride 0.18%, sodium chloride 0.9%, and water for injection, at concentrations of 0.25–1 mg/mL. Aminophylline is also stable for 24 hours at 25°C at 29 µg/mL concentration in TPN solution, and for 14 and seven days at 8°C and 37°C, respectively, in CADD-Plus infusion cassettes at 5 mg/mL or 12.5 mg/mL concentration.

On exposure to air, aminophylline solutions gradually liberate free theophylline which is less soluble. Solutions should be inspected for crystallisation prior to use and should not be used if crystals are present.

Many physical incompatibilities have been reported due to the high pH of the aminophylline injection (pH 8.6–9.0). For this reason, information on physical compatibility must be interpreted with care.

References

1. Reynolds JEF, editor. Martindale: the extra pharmacopoeia, 31st edition. London: The Pharmaceutical Press, 1996: 1651-2.
2. Trissel LA. Handbook on injectable drugs, 9th edition. Bethesda, MD: American Society of Health-System Pharmacists Inc, 1996: 55-66.
3. Wermeling DP, et al. Osmolality of small-volume intravenous admixtures. Am J Hosp Pharm 1985; 42: 1739-44.
4. Romankiewicz JA, et al. Medications not to be refrigerated. Am J Hosp Pharm 1979; 36: 1541-5.
5. McEvoy GK, editor. American hospital formulary service drug information 1997. Bethesda, MD: American Society of Health-System Pharmacists Inc, 1997: 2796-803.
6. Adams PS, Haines-Nutt RF, Ross ID. The stability of aminophylline in intravenous infusion solutions. Proc Guild 1988; 25: 41-4.
7. Parker EA. Aminophylline intravenous. Am J Hosp Pharm 1970; 27: 67-9.
8. Edward M. pH – an important factor in the compatibility of additives in intravenous therapy. Am J Hosp Pharm 1967; 24: 440-9.
9. Simmons A, Allwood MC. Sorption to plastic syringes of drugs administered by syringe pump. J Clin Hosp Pharm 1981; 6: 71-3.
10. Nahata MC, Morosco RS, Hipple TF. Stability of aminophylline in bacteriostatic water for injection stored in plastic syringes at two temperatures. Am J Hosp Pharm 1992; 49: 2962-3.
11. Kirk B, Sprake JM. Stability of aminophylline. Br J Intraven Ther 1982; 3(11): 4-8.

12. Taylor A. A physical compatibility study of clarithromycin injection with other commonly used injectable drugs. Pharm in Pract 1997; 7(9): 473-6.

13. Stewart JT, Warren FW, King AD. Stability of ranitidine hydrochloride and seven medications. Am J Hosp Pharm 1994; 51: 1802-7.

14. Stewart JT, Warren FW, Johnson SM. Stability of cefuroxime sodium and aminophylline or theophylline. Am J Hosp Pharm 1994; 51: 809-11.

15. Johnson CE, et al. Stability and compatibility of fluconazole and aminophylline in intravenous admixtures. Am J Hosp Pharm 1993; 50: 703-6.

16. Driscoll DF, et al. Parenteral nutrient admixtures as drug vehicles: theory and practice in the critical care setting. Drug Intell Clin Pharm 1991; 25: 276-82.

17. Johnson CE, et al. Compatibility of aminophylline and methylprednisolone sodium succinate intravenous admixtures. Am J Hosp Pharm 1986; 43:1482-5.

Prepared by

Melanie Priston

Amoxycillin

Approved Name
Amoxycillin

UK Proprietary Name
Almodan (Berk)
Amoxil (Bencard)

Other Names
Amoxicillin.

Product Details
Glass vials containing the equivalent of 250 mg, 500 mg, or 1 g of amoxycillin. The injection consists of the sodium salt as a freeze-dried powder. The sodium content is 3.3 mmol/1 g vial.[1]

Preparation of Injection
The content of each vial is reconstituted by dissolving in water for injection using 5 mL for each 250 mg of amoxycillin.

If more accurate reconstitution is required (e.g. for paediatric use) the displacement value is 0.8 mL/g.[1] For infusion, the resulting solution may be diluted with sodium chloride 0.9%. Alternatively, using a suitable reconstitution device the vial may be reconstituted using the infusion bag.[1]

Administration
May be administered by intravenous injection over 3–4 minutes, or by intravenous infusion over 30–60 minutes in sodium chloride 0.9%.[1]

Stability in Practice
Amoxycillin sodium 5% is much less stable in all infusion solutions than at lower concentrations of 1% or 2%.[2,3] Solutions undergo both hydrolysis and aminolysis, with hydrolysis assuming greater importance as concentration decreases and pH rises.[2]

Published Information Amoxycillin 1% and 2% stored at room temperature has been shown to be stable for up to eight hours (less than 10% loss of activity) in sodium chloride 0.9%, whilst an amoxycillin 5% solution showed 10% loss of activity after three hours. In glucose 5%, amoxycillin solution showed more than 10% loss of activity after less than two hours.[3]

For refrigerated or frozen solutions, the rate of degradation increases as temperature rises, but it also increases below 0°C.[4] Amoxycillin sodium 10 mg/mL in sodium chloride 0.9% was stable for 10.5 days at 0°C (unfrozen) and 14 hours when frozen at -19°C. When the same concentration in glucose 5% was studied, stability was 12.5 hours at 0°C and 8.4 hours at -19°C.[5]

The rate of freezing and thawing could account for losses of amoxycillin in PVC minibags due to a saturated solution being present during thawing.[3,6]

Unpublished Information The chemical stability of amoxycillin was investigated at 5°C in the following concentrations and diluents and demonstrated at least 90% of declared potency for the following times.

Diluent	Amoxycillin 1%	Amoxycillin 5%
Glucose 5%	7 hours	2 hours
Sodium chloride 0.9%	3 days	4 hours
Water for injection	4 days	6 hours

Incompatibilities Amoxycillin has been reported to be physically or chemically incompatible with the following drug substances: aminoglycosides; ciprofloxacin; and perfloxacin.[7]

Compatibilities Specialist references should be consulted for specific compatibility information.[7,8]

Comments
Both published and unpublished work indicates that the stability of amoxycillin is much greater at a concentration of 1% than 5%. A 1% solution of amoxycillin in sodium chloride 0.9% shows a stability of no more than three days at 5°C. However, at room temperature stability is much less, and this must be taken into account when considering product expiry unless the cold chain can be guaranteed. Freezing amoxycillin does not improve the product shelf-life.

References

1. ABPI. Compendium of data sheets and summaries of product characteristics 1996-1997. London: Datapharm Publications Ltd, 1996: 120-1.
2. Cook B, Hill SA, Lynn B. The stability of amoxycillin sodium in intravenous infusion fluids. J Clin Hosp Pharm 1982; 7: 245-50.
3. Lynn B. The stability and administration of intravenous penicillins. Br J Intraven Ther 1981; 2(3): 22-39.
4. Concannon J, et al. Stability of aqueous solutions of amoxicillin sodium in the frozen and liquid states. Am J Hosp Pharm 1986; 43: 3027-30.
5. McDonald C, et al. The stability of amoxycillin sodium in normal saline and glucose (5%) solutions in the liquid and frozen states. J Clin Pharm Ther 1989; 14: 45-52.
6. McDonald C, et al. Freezing rates of 50 mL infusion bags and some implications for drug stability as shown with amoxycillin. Aust J Hosp Pharm 1989; 19: 194-7.
7. Trissel LA. Handbook on injectable drugs, 9th edition. Bethesda, MD: American Society of Health-System Pharmacists Inc, 1996: 1113-5.
8. Janknegt R, et al. Quinolones and penicillins incompatibility. DICP Ann Pharmacother 1989; 23: 91-2.

Prepared by

Christine Clarke

Amphotericin

Approved Name
Amphotericin B

UK Proprietary Name
Fungizone (Bristol-Myers Squibb)

Other Names
—

Product Details
Glass vials containing a yellow fluffy powder of amphotericin 50000 units (50 mg). Vials also contain desoxycholic acid and sodium phosphates.[1] A 3% injection has a pH of 6–8.[2] In glucose 5%, a 0.1 mg/mL solution has an osmolality of 256 mosmol/kg.[3] Sodium content is less than 0.5 mmol/50 mg.

Preparation of Injection
Water for injection (10 mL) should be added to the contents of one vial and shaken to produce a clear colloidal solution containing amphotericin 5 mg/mL. This solution should then be diluted (1:50) with glucose 5% (pH greater than 4.2) to produce an amphotericin 0.1 mg/mL infusion. Commercially available glucose 5% infusions usually have a pH greater than 4.2; however, the pH can be suitably adjusted before the amphotericin is added, by adding 1 mL or 2 mL of a phosphate buffer to the glucose infusion.[1]

Administration
Amphotericin should be administered by infusion over a period of up to six hours. If in-line filtration is required, a filter with a mean pore diameter of not less than 1 µm should be used so that the colloidal dispersion can pass through.[1]

Stability in Practice
The major route of degradation of amphotericin, in aqueous solution, appears to be epoxidation and *trans-cis* isomerisation. Dilute solutions are light sensitive. Amphotericin is inactivated at low pH.[2]

In aqueous solution at pH 4–8, degradation has been shown to follow first-order kinetics. Maximum stability and optimum clarity of amphotericin, at 37°C in the presence of phosphate buffer, occurs at pH 5–7.[2]

When diluted in the vial with water for injection, amphotericin is chemically stable when stored for 24 hours at room temperature or one week if refrigerated.[1] When diluted in PVC bags, studies have shown little degradation after 35 days at 4°C[4] or five days at 25°C when protected from light.[5]

Published Information Amphotericin has been reported to be incompatible with sodium chloride 0.9%, a precipitate forming within two hours with the loss of 43% of the initial amount of drug within this time. In the same study, amphotericin was reported to be stable for at least 48 hours at 25°C with glucose 5%.[6]

An early study[7] suggested a three day shelf-life for 100 mg of amphotericin in 1000 mL of glucose 5% or six weeks at 5°C, when stored in glass. This has been confirmed by other work[4,5] which showed that amphotericin in glucose 5%, stored in PVC bags, was stable for up to 35 days when stored at 4°C and five days when stored at 25°C protected from light.

The stability of amphotericin in higher strengths of glucose has also been investigated. Amphotericin 0.1 mg/mL was found to be stable for at least 24 hours when stored at 15–25°C, protected from light, in glucose 5%, 10%, 15%, and 20% in 50 mL PVC bags.[8] Amphotericin stability has also been studied in polyolefin containers at the concentrations commonly used for administration through a central venous line (amphotericin 60, 80, and 100 mg in 50 mL of glucose 5%). At these concentrations, in this container, no significant degradation was seen at either 6°C or 25°C when stored for up to 36 hours.[9]

Nephrotoxicity is a complication for patients treated with long courses of amphotericin. However, the administration of amphotericin in parenteral fat emulsions has been said to reduce the risk of nephrotoxicity[10] although this work has been challenged[11] on the basis that the mixture separated into two phases within four hours of mixing. Despite this separation, it was claimed that the dispersion when re-suspended by shaking was stable for four days at 20–25°C when exposed to fluorescent light or seven days when protected from fluorescent light or at 4–8°C.[12] However, it has been suggested[11] that the extraction and assay technique used may well have caused re-dispersion and re-dissolution of the amphotericin thus leading to falsely high results. Other work[13] shows that although amphotericin 45 mg in 500 mL of lipid was stable for up to one hour, the concentration of amphotericin fell to 56% of the expected amount within six hours. It was concluded that amphotericin was unstable in the lipid emulsion and that any reduced toxicity might be due to inadequate dosing. S*ee also* below.

Unpublished Information   Amphotericin 2 g/L in lipid 20% emulsion has been said to be unstable due to the formation of a yellow precipitate.[14]

Amphotericin 0.2 mg/mL in glucose 5% was reported to be stable in an elastomeric infusion device for 24 hours at room temperature or 10 days if refrigerated. However, it was noted that amphotericin had the potential to precipitate, depending upon the concentration, pH and storage conditions.[15]

Incompatibilities   Amphotericin solutions have been reported to be physically or chemically incompatible with the following drug substances: amikacin sulphate; ampicillin; benzylpenicillin; calcium chloride; calcium gluconate; carbenicillin sodium; chlorpromazine hydrochloride; chlortetracycline hydrochloride; cimetidine hydrochloride; diphenhydramine hydrochloride; dopamine hydrochloride; foscarnet sodium; gentamicin sulphate; kanamycin sulphate; lignocaine hydrochloride; metaraminol tartrate; methyldopa hydrochloride; nitrofurantoin sodium; oxytetracycline hydrochloride; polymixin B sulphate; potassium chloride; procaine hydrochloride; prochlorperazine mesylate; ranitidine hydrochloride; sodium calcium edetate; sodium chloride; tetracycline hydrochloride; verapamil hydrochloride; and viomycin sulphate.[2,3,16]

Comments

In common clinical practice, amphotericin in glucose 5% is stable for up to 35 days when stored at 4°C and protected from light. Information on physical compatibility must be interpreted with care, particularly compatibility with lipid emulsions.

References

1. ABPI. Compendium of data sheets and summaries of product characteristics 1996-1997. London: Datapharm Publications Ltd, 1996: 1135-6.

2. Lund W, editor. The pharmaceutical codex: principles and practice of pharmaceutics, 12th edition. London: The Pharmaceutical Press, 1994: 731-3.

3. Trissel LA. Handbook on injectable drugs, 9th edition. Bethesda, MD: American Society of Health-System Pharmacists Inc, 1996: 74-9.

4. Mitrano FP, et al. Chemical and visual stability of amphotericin B in 5% dextrose injection stored at 4°C for 35 days. Am J Hosp Pharm 1991; 48: 2635-7.

5. Lee MD, et al. Stability of amphotericin B in 5% dextrose injection stored at 4 or 25°C for 120 hours. Am J Hosp Pharm 1994; 51: 394-6.

6. Jurgens RW, DeLuca PP, Papadimitriou D. Compatibility of amphotericin B with certain large-volume parenterals. Am J Hosp Pharm 1981; 38: 377-8.

7. Gallelli JF. Stability studies of drugs used in intravenous solutions: part one. Am J Hosp Pharm 1967; 24: 425-33.

8. Wiest DB, et al. Stability of amphotericin B in four concentrations of dextrose injection. Am J Hosp Pharm 1991; 48: 2430-33.

9. Kintzel PE, Kennedy PE. Stability of amphotericin B in 5% dextrose injection at concentrations used for administration through a central venous line. Am J Hosp Pharm 1991; 48: 283-5.

10. Chavanet PY, et al. Trial of glucose versus fat emulsion in preparation of amphotericin for use in HIV infected patients with candidiasis. Br Med J 1992; 305: 921-5.

11. Kintzel PE. Amphotericin B in fat emulsion. Am J Health-Syst Pharm 1996; 53: 2701.

12. Lopez RM, et al. Stability of amphotericin B in an extemporaneously prepared i.v. fat emulsion. Am J Health-Syst Pharm 1996; 53: 2724-7.

13. Ericsson O. Amphotericin B is incompatible with lipid emulsions. Ann Pharmacother 1996; 30: 298.

14. Grassby PF. Personal communication, 1996.

15. Block Medical Inc. Personal communication, 1996.

16. Reynolds JEF, editor. Martindale: the extra pharmacopoeia, 31st edition. London: The Pharmaceutical Press, 1996: 398-402.

Prepared by

Sandra Harding and Frank Haines-Nutt

Ampicillin

Approved Name
Ampicillin sodium

UK Proprietary Name
Amfipen (Yamanouchi Ltd)
Penbritin (SmithKline Beecham)

Other Names
—

Product Details
Available as glass vials for reconstitution containing 250 mg or 500 mg of ampicillin as ampicillin sodium.[1] A 10% injection has a pH of 8–10. The osmolality of a 100 mg/mL solution is 602 mosmol/kg.[2] Ampicillin is compatible with PVC infusion bags.[3] Sodium content: 0.73 mmol/250 mg; 1.47 mmol/500 mg.

Preparation of Injection
For intramuscular injection, 1.5 mL of water for injection should be added to either a 250 mg or 500 mg vial.

For intravenous injection, a 250 mg vial should be diluted with 5 mL of water for injection and a 500 mg vial with 10 mL.

For intraperitoneal and intrapleural injection, a 500 mg vial should be diluted with 5–10 mL of water for injection.

For intra-articular injection, a 500 mg vial should be diluted with 5 mL of water for injection or sterile 0.5% procaine hydrochloride solution.

Administration
Ampicillin may be administered by a variety of routes, *see* above, including intramuscular injection, slow intravenous injection over 3–4 minutes, and intravenous infusion. Suitable infusion solutions include: glucose 5%; glucose 4% with sodium chloride 0.18%; sodium chloride 0.9%; and water for injection.

Stability in Practice
In dilute aqueous solution, ampicillin degrades primarily through hydrolysis although at higher concentrations polymerisation also occurs. Early sources suggested a shelf-life of approximately seven days for a 1% solution in sodium chloride 0.9% and 24 hours for a 5% solution.[4] However, more recent sources suggest a shelf-life of between 3–5 days at 5°C, for a 1% or 2% solution, based on a 10% loss in potency.[2] Other recent reports suggest a shelf-life of between 12–48 hours for unbuffered ampicillin solutions.[5-7]

The manufacturer states that once reconstituted, ampicillin solutions for injection should be used immediately. Infusions may be refrigerated (2–8°C) and used within 24 hours of preparation. However, solutions containing glucose or other carbohydrates should be used within one hour.[1]

Published Information   The stability of ampicillin is concentration dependent and decreases rapidly at higher concentrations. Sodium chloride 0.9% appears to be the most suitable diluent for ampicillin sodium. Storage temperature and solution pH affects the stability.[4] Stability is also greatly decreased in glucose solutions.[1,2]

Much of the early work on ampicillin stability depended on non-specific assay methods.[8-10] Despite this, one study showed an ampicillin degradation of 3.3% after 24 hours at 5°C[10] while in another study[8] it was reported that at a concentration of 0.5–4% in sodium chloride 0.9% approximately 1–6% loss of ampicillin potency occurred within 25 hours in a refrigerator. In other studies, approximately 3–4% ampicillin degradation was reported at 5°C and 12–18% at 25°C in 24 hours for a 2% solution.[11] Using a stability indicating assay, for 1% and 2% ampicillin solutions in sodium chloride 0.9%, a 10% reduction in ampicillin content after 48 hours at 4°C was reported, with a similar loss of ampicillin in less than 24 hours at 25°C.[7] These results agree quite closely with another study,[6] where a shelf-life of 48 hours for a 1% ampicillin solution in sodium chloride 0.9% stored in PVC bags at 4°C, was reported. At room temperature a shelf-life of six hours was suggested.

For higher concentrations, such as 5% ampicillin in syringes, a shelf-life of 24 hours has been suggested at 4°C, and eight hours at 20°C. At 10% concentration, 10% degradation occurred in 12 hours at

4°C. This report is consistent with another study which showed a 36% loss of ampicillin in two days for a refrigerated 12.5% solution in water for injection.[12]

Studies on unbuffered solutions indicated that ampicillin was too unstable to recommend storage after reconstitution, even in sodium chloride 0.9%, with a maximum shelf-life of 24 hours after preparation. However, buffered solutions were found to be more stable. Studies on ampicillin buffered with potassium acid phosphate injection 13.6% (1 mL added to 250 mg of ampicillin in 50 mL sodium chloride 0.9%) suggested the shelf-life could be extended to 12 days. If 2 mL of buffer was added to 500 mg ampicillin in 100 mL of sodium chloride 0.9% the solution was stable for six days.[5]

When stored in an elastomeric infusion device it was reported that 2% ampicillin in sodium chloride 0.9% was stable for eight hours at 25°C and three days at 5°C; similar stability to that in glass.[13]

Ampicillin is reported to be extremely unstable in glucose 5%, at any temperature, with degradation of up to 90% in four hours.[8,9]

Unpublished Information In studies of ampicillin stability at various temperatures (including refrigeration) in compound sodium lactate and glucose 5%, up to 36% ampicillin degradation was said to have occurred in 24 hours. Reconstitution with these diluents was therefore not recommended.

Ampicillin sodium 20 mg/mL in sodium chloride 0.9% was reported to be stable in an elastomeric infusion device for eight hours at room temperature or three days if refrigerated.[14]

Incompatibilities Ampicillin sodium solutions have been reported to be physically or chemically incompatible with the following drug substances: acetylcysteine; adrenaline; amikacin sulphate; amphotericin; atropine sulphate; calcium chloride; calcium gluconate; chloramphenicol sodium succinate; chlorpromazine hydrochloride; chlortetracycline; clindamycin phosphate; dopamine hydrochloride; erythromycin ethyl succinate; erythromycin lactobionate; gentamicin sulphate; heparin; hydralazine hydrochloride; hydrocortisone sodium succinate; kanamycin sulphate; lincomycin hydrochloride; metoclopramide; metaraminol tartrate; metronidazole; noradrenaline; novobiocin; oxytetracycline hydrochloride; pentobarbitone; phenobarbitone; prochlorperazine mesylate and edisylate; polymyxin B sulphate; protein hydrolysate; sodium bicarbonate; sulphafurazole; suxamethonium; tetracycline hydrochloride; thiopentone; and vitamin B and C solutions.[2,15,16]

Compatibilities Specialist references should be consulted for details of compatibility data.[2] Information on physical compatibility should be interpreted with care.

Intravenous admixtures of ampicillin and aztreonam have been investigated in glucose 5% and sodium chloride 0.9% infusions stored at 25°C for 48 hours and 4°C for seven days. Stability was assessed for pH changes, microscopically for particulates, and by HPLC. The pH was influenced by the concentration of the drugs and stability was influenced by the pH. No evidence of a direct reaction between the drugs was seen but stability was affected by pH changes produced by the two drugs. In sodium chloride 0.9% infusion, ampicillin 5 mg/mL and 10 mg/mL with aztreonam 10 mg/mL and 20 mg/mL, was reported to be stable for 48 hours at 25°C or seven days at 4°C. In glucose 5%, storage should not exceed 24 hours at 25°C or 48 hours at 4°C.[17]

Comments

Ampicillin 1% or 2% in sodium chloride 0.9% is stable for up to 48 hours when stored at 5°C although even this is disputed by some authors. At higher concentrations, such as that used in syringes, the shelf-life for 10% degradation is less than 24 hours when refrigerated.

References

1. ABPI. Compendium of data sheets and summaries of product characteristics 1996-1997. London: Datapharm Publications Ltd, 1996: 118.
2. Trissel LA. Handbook on injectable drugs, 9th edition. Bethesda, MD: American Society of Health-System Pharmacists Inc, 1996: 79-94.
3. Kowaluk EA, et al. Interactions between drugs and polyvinyl chloride infusion bags. Am J Hosp Pharm 1981; 38: 1308-14.
4. The pharmaceutical codex, 11th edition. London: The Pharmaceutical Press, 1979: 42-44.
5. Allwood MC, Brown PW. Stability of ampicillin infusions in unbuffered and buffered saline. Int J Pharmaceutics 1993; 97: 219-22.
6. Adams P. The stability of reconstituted ampicillin injection in syringes and minibags. Pharm J 1992; 249(Suppl): HS21.
7. James MJ, Riley CM. Stability of intravenous admixtures of aztreonam and ampicillin. Am J Hosp Pharm 1985; 42: 1095-1100.

8. Hiranaka PK, Frazier AG, Gallelli JF. Stability of sodium ampicillin in aqueous solutions. Am J Hosp Pharm 1972; 29: 321-2.

9. Gallelli JF, MacLowry JD, Skolaut MW. Stability of antibiotics in parenteral solutions. Am J Hosp Pharm 1969; 26: 630-5.

10. Savello DR, Shangraw RF. Stability of sodium ampicillin solutions in the frozen and liquid states. Am J Hosp Pharm 1971; 28: 754-9.

11. Warren E, et al. Stability of ampicillin in intravenous solutions. Mayo Clinic Proc 1972; 47: 34-5.

12. Ahmed ST, Parkinson R. The stability of drugs in pre-filled syringes: flucloxacillin, ampicillin, cefuroxime, cefotaxime and ceftazidime. Hosp Pharm Pract 1992; 2: 285-9.

13. Allen LV, et al. Stability of 14 drugs in the latex reservoir of an elastomeric infusion device. Am J Health-Syst Pharm 1996; 53: 2740-3.

14. Block Medical Inc. Personal communication, 1996.

15. Reynolds JEF, editor. Martindale: the extra pharmacopoeia, 31st edition. London: The Pharmaceutical Press, 1996: 172-4.

16. Lund W, editor. The pharmaceutical codex: principles and practice of pharmaceutics, 12th edition. London: The Pharmaceutical Press, 1994: 733-9.

17. James MJ, Riley CM. Stability of intravenous admixtures of aztreonam and ampicillin. Am J Hosp Pharm 1985; 42: 1095-1100.

Prepared by

Sandra Harding and Frank Haines-Nutt

Aztreonam

Approved Name
Aztreonam

UK Proprietary Name
Azactam for Injection (Bristol-Myers Squibb)

Other Names
—

Product Details
Clear glass 15 mL vials containing 500 mg, 1 g, or 2 g, of sterile aztreonam as a white to off-white powder. Each vial also contains 780 mg L-arginine per gram of aztreonam.[1] Aztreonam is soluble 10 mg/mL in water; the pH of the injection is 4.5–7.5 when reconstituted in aqueous solution.[2] Aztreonam injection is sodium free.

Preparation of Injection
The contents of each vial are reconstituted with water for injection, and immediately shaken vigorously. The resultant solution may vary in colour from colourless through a light straw-yellow to amber colour, depending on concentration and diluent. A slight pink tinge may develop on standing; this colour does not indicate loss of potency.

Vials are reconstituted with water for injection as in the table below.

Size	For intramuscular injection	For intravenous injection
500 mg	1.5 mL	3.0 mL
1 g	3.0 mL	3.0 mL
2 g	–	3.0 mL

If more accurate reconstitution is required (e.g. for paediatric use) the following powder displacement value may be used: 0.4 mL/500 mg.[3]

For intravenous administration, the solution must be further diluted with at least 50 mL of infusion fluid per gram of aztreonam, to a final concentration of less than 2%. Suitable infusion solutions include: compound sodium lactate; glucose 5%; mannitol 5% or 10%; Ringer's solution; and sodium chloride 0.9%.[1]

Administration
Aztreonam 0.5–1 g may be administered intramuscularly every 8–12 hours. Alternatively, injections of 0.5–2 g may be infused every 6–8 hours, depending on the nature and severity of infection. Infusions are given over 20–60 minutes.

Stability in Practice
The unreconstituted injection should be stored at room temperature (15–25°C); maximum storage temperature is 40°C. It is recommended that the injection is used immediately after reconstitution, although storage in a refrigerator (2–7°C) for 24 hours may be permitted.[1]

In aqueous media, the decomposition of aztreonam follows first-order kinetics, with hydrolysis of the beta-lactam ring being the most important degradation pathway. At pH values greater than pH 6, specific base catalysis occurs. In the range pH 2–5 isomerisation of the aminothiazole oxime side-chain is the predominant reaction. The drug is inactivated in solutions with a pH below pH 1 or greater than pH 8.[4,5] Optimum stability is in the range pH 5–7, with minimum decomposition rates at pH 6.

Published Information   The stability of aztreonam in infusion solutions has been investigated using degradation sensitive HPLC techniques.

The antimicrobial activity of heated solutions of aztreonam against two strains of *Staphylococcus aureus*, two strains of *Escherichia coli* and one strain of *Bacilus subtilis* demonstrated some retention of activity after autoclaving at 121°C for 15 minutes or heating at 56°C for 30 minutes.[6]

Following reconstitution with water for injection and addition to glucose 5% or sodium chloride 0.9% solution, aztreonam was found to be stable for 48 hours at 15–30°C, or for seven days when refrigerated at 2–8°C.[5]

Solutions containing aztreonam 1 g/50 mL or 2 g/100 mL, in sodium chloride 0.9% infusion in PVC minibags were stored at -20°C, 4°C, 25°C, and 37°C for 120 days. Stability was investigated using HPLC and bioassay techniques. From the results obtained, a shelf-life of 60 days in a refrigerator was assigned, although the time for 10% decomposition at 4°C was calculated to be 267 days, and at 25°C, 37.5 days.[7]

At concentrations of 20 mg/mL (2%) or less, aztreonam is reported to be physically and chemically stable for 48 hours at 15–30°C or seven days when refrigerated at 2–8°C in the common infusion solutions e.g. glucose 5% or sodium chloride 0.9%. At concentrations greater than 2%, aztreonam is reported to be stable for 48 hours at 2–8°C in water for injection or sodium chloride 0.9%. Solutions above 2% concentration in other solutions should be used immediately.[2]

The stability of aztreonam 60 mg/mL in water for injection in a PVC portable pump reservoir was investigated. No significant losses were observed after six months at -20°C or eight days at 5°C. During simulated pumping for 24 hours at 37°C a 3.6% decrease in aztreonam concentration was recorded.[8]

Aztreonam solutions frozen at -20°C are reported to be stable for 90 days. When thawed and stored at room temperature the solution should be used within 24 hours. Those solutions that have been thawed and stored at 2–8°C should be used within 72 hours.[2]

Unpublished Information Aztreonam in a concentration range of 13.33–26.66 mg/mL in sodium chloride 0.9% was reported to be stable in an elastomeric infusion device for seven days at either room temperature or in a refrigerator.[9]

At a concentration between 20–30 mg/mL aztreonam was found to be stable for 14 days at room temperature in an elastomeric infusion chamber.[9]

Incompatibilities Aztreonam solutions have been reported to be incompatible with the following drug substances: amsacrine; metronidazole; nafcillin; and vancomycin hydrochloride.

Compatibilities Specialist references should be consulted for details of compatibility information. Information on physical compatibility should be interpreted with care.

Intravenous admixtures of aztreonam and ampicillin have been investigated in glucose 5% and sodium chloride 0.9% infusions stored at 25°C for 48 hours and at 4°C for seven days. Stability was assessed for pH changes, microscopically for particulates, and by HPLC. The pH was influenced by the concentration of the drugs and stability was influenced by the pH. No evidence of a direct reaction between the drugs was seen but stability was affected by pH changes produced by the two drugs. In sodium chloride 0.9% infusion, ampicillin 5 mg/mL and 10 mg/mL with aztreonam 10 mg/mL and 20 mg/mL, was reported to be stable for 48 hours at 25°C, or seven days at 4°C. In glucose 5%, storage should not exceed 24 hours at 25°C or 48 hours at 4°C.[5]

A similar study found clindamycin phosphate 3 mg/mL and 6 mg/mL in glucose 5% and sodium chloride 0.9% infusion with aztreonam 10 mg/mL and 20 mg/mL, to be stable for 48 hours at 22–23°C, or seven days at 4°C.[10]

Aztreonam was found to be chemically and physically compatible with ranitidine for at least four hours during simulated Y-site administration.[11]

Compatibility has been demonstrated in glucose 5% and sodium chloride 0.9%, by an HPLC method, over 48 hours at 25°C or seven days at 4°C with the following intravenous injections: cephazolin; clindamycin phosphate; and tobramycin.[10,12,13]

Compatibility has also been demonstrated by an HPLC method over 12 hours at 25°C or seven days at 4°C with cefoxitin, and for eight hours at 25°C or 24 hours at 4°C with gentamicin[12] although another study indicated that cefoxitin content in solutions containing aztreonam in glucose 5% or sodium chloride 0.9% decreased by more than 10% within 48 hours at 25°C, and within seven days at 4°C.[14] No loss of aztreonam was detected.[14]

Aztreonam 10 mg/mL with ampicillin 20 mg/mL and sulbactam 10 mg/mL in sodium chloride 0.9% was found to be stable for up to 30 hours at room temperature and 94 hours at 5°C.[15]

Comments

—

References

1. ABPI. Compendium of data sheets and summaries of product characteristics 1996-1997. London: Datapharm Publications Ltd, 1996: 1130-1.
2. McEvoy GK, editor. American hospital formulary service drug information 1997. Bethesda, MD: American Society of Health-System Pharmacists Inc, 1997: 186-94.
3. Mulholland P. Displacement values of powder injections. Pharm J 1993; 251: 14-5.
4. Méndez R, Alemany T, Martín-Villacorta J. Stability in aqueous solution of two monocyclic ß-lactam antibiotics: aztreonam and nocardicin A. Chem Pharm Bull (Tokyo) 1992; 40: 3222-7.

5. James MJ, Riley CM. Stability of intravenous admixtures of aztreonam and ampicillin. Am J Hosp Pharm 1985; 42: 1095-1100.
6. Traub WH, Leonhard B. Heat stability of the antimicrobial activity of sixty-two antibacterial agents. J Antimicrob Chemother 1995; 35: 149-54.
7. McLaughlin JP, Simpson C. The stability of reconstituted aztreonam. Br J Pharm Pract 1990; 12: 328-34.
8. Vinks AAT, et al. Stability of aztreonam in a portable pump reservoir used for home intravenous antibiotic treatment. Pharm World Sci 1996; 18: 74-7.
9. Block Medical Inc. Personal communication, 1996.
10. James MJ, Riley CM. Stability of intravenous admixtures of aztreonam and clindamycin phosphate. Am J Hosp Pharm 1985; 42: 1984-6.
11. Inagaki K, et al. Stability of ranitidine hydrochloride with aztreonam, ceftazidime, or piperacillin sodium during simulated Y-site administration. Am J Hosp Pharm 1992; 49: 2769-72.
12. Marble DA, Bosso JA, Townsend RJ. Stability of clindamycin phosphate with aztreonam, ceftazidime sodium, ceftriaxone sodium, or piperacillin sodium in two intravenous solutions. Am J Hosp Pharm 1986; 43: 1732-6.
13. Riley CM, James MJ. Stability of intravenous admixtures containing aztreonam and cefazolin. Am J Hosp Pharm 1986; 43: 925-7.
14. Bell RG, et al. Stability of intravenous admixtures of aztreonam and cefoxitin, gentamicin, metronidazole, or tobramycin. Am J Hosp Pharm 1986; 43: 1444-53.
15. Belliveau PP, Nightingale CH, Quintiliani R. Stability of aztreonam and ampicillin sodium-sulbactam sodium in 0.9% sodium chloride injection. Am J Hosp Pharm 1994; 51: 901-4.

Prepared by

Tim Sizer

Benzylpenicillin Sodium

Approved Name
Benzylpenicillin sodium

UK Proprietary Name
Crystapen (Britannia Pharmaceuticals Ltd)

Other Names
Penicillin G.

Product Details
Vials containing 600 mg (1 mega unit) of benzylpenicillin sodium as a white crystalline powder. The sodium content is 38.6 mg/600 mg (1.68 mmol).[1] The pH of the reconstituted injection varies depending upon the pH of the diluent. An aqueous 10% benzylpenicillin sodium solution has a pH of 5.5–7.5.[2]

Preparation of Injection
The content of each vial is reconstituted by dissolving in sodium chloride 0.9% or water for injection. Recommended dilutions are: for intramuscular injection, dissolve in 1.6–2 mL of water for injection; for intravenous injection, dissolve in 4–10 mL of water for injection; for intravenous infusion, dissolve in at least 10 mL of sodium chloride 0.9%.[1] Infusions may be further diluted with glucose 5% or sodium chloride 0.9%.

If more accurate reconstitution is required (e.g. for paediatric use) the following powder displacement value may be used: 0.4 mL/600 mg.[3]

Administration
Benzylpenicillin sodium may be administered by intramuscular injection, intravenous injection, or intravenous infusion. Other routes of administration, such as intrathecal injection may also be used.[1]

Stability in Practice
The manufacturer states that the reconstituted injection, or the injection after dilution in the recommended infusions, is stable at 2–8°C for up to 24 hours.[1]

Published Information The chemical stability of benzylpenicillin sodium was investigated in sodium chloride 0.9% stored in 50 mL PVC infusion bags after reconstitution of the injection with either water for injection or a citrate buffer. Drug concentrations were 12 mg/mL and 48 mg/mL for the unbuffered solutions and 12 mg/mL for the buffered solution. Storage was at 5°C for up to 28 days. No details of light protection were provided. Analysis was by stability indicating HPLC assay. Results indicated a shelf-life of 48 hours (maximum acceptable loss of 10%) for unbuffered solutions. For citrate buffered solutions (pH 6.5–7.5) results indicated a shelf-life of 28 days (loss of 5.5%).[4]

Benzylpenicillin 12 mg/mL in sodium chloride 0.9% in 100 mL PVC minibags was found to be stable, by HPLC assay methods, for two days in a refrigerator or 24 hours at room temperature, protected from light.[5]

The chemical stability of benzylpenicillin sodium was investigated in sodium chloride 0.9% stored in polypropylene syringes after reconstitution of the injection with either water for injection or a citrate buffer. Drug concentrations were 54 mg/mL, 107 mg/mL, and 144 mg/mL. Storage was at 5°C for up to 14 days. No details of light protection were provided. Analysis was by stability indicating HPLC assay. Results indicated a shelf-life of 48 hours (maximum acceptable loss of 10%) for unbuffered solutions. For citrate buffered solutions (pH 6.8) results indicated a shelf-life of at least 14 days (loss of less than 5%).[6]

The stability of benzylpenicillin sodium in pre-filled PVC portable pump reservoirs was studied during simulated in-use conditions. Benzylpenicillin at a concentration of 180000 units/mL was filled into a 15 mL reservoir, stored at -20°C for 30 days, thawed to refrigerator temperature (5°C) for four days and then connected to a pump for a 24 hour pumping cycle at 37°C. Results indicated that benzylpenicillin should not be administered for more than 12 hours after such a cycle of freezing and thawing.[7]

Unpublished Information Benzylpenicillin potassium 6 mg/mL in glucose 5% was reported to be stable in an elastomeric infusion device for 24 hours at room temperature or refrigerated, and for 30 days when frozen.

Incompatibilities Incompatibility or loss of activity of benzylpenicillin (as either the sodium or potassium salt) has been reported with the following drug substances: aminacrine hydrochloride; aminophylline; amphotericin; ascorbic acid; cephaloridine; cephalothin sodium; chlorpromazine hydrochloride; cysteine; ephedrine; erythromycin ethyl succinate; heparin sodium; hydroxyzine hydrochloride; iodine/iodides; lincomycin hydrochloride; metaraminol tartrate; metoclopramide hydrochloride; noradrenaline acid tartrate; oxytetracycline hydrochloride; phenytoin sodium; pentobarbitone sodium; procaine hydrochloride; prochlorperazine salts; promazine hydrochloride; promethazine hydrochloride; resorcinol; sodium bicarbonate; streptomycin sulphate; tetracycline hydrochloride; thiamine hydrochloride; thiopentone sodium; trometamol; and vancomycin hydrochloride.[2]

Compatibilities Specialist references should be consulted for details of compatibility information. Information on physical compatibility should be interpreted with care.

Comments

Reconstituted benzylpenicillin sodium is relatively stable in solutions buffered to pH 6.5–7.5. Unbuffered solutions of benzylpenicillin sodium in sodium chloride 0.9% stored at 5°C in PVC infusion bags or polypropylene syringes should be administered within 48 hours of preparation. Citrate buffered solutions of benzylpenicillin sodium in sodium chloride 0.9% at pH 6.5–7.5 may be stored at 5°C for 28 days in PVC bags and for 14 days in polypropylene syringes. Degradation rates have been found to be independent of concentration. Stability is pH dependent with an optimum of pH 6.8.[8]

References

1. ABPI. Compendium of data sheets and summaries of product characteristics 1996-1997. London: Datapharm Publications Ltd, 1996: 182.
2. Lund W, editor. The pharmaceutical codex: principles and practice of pharmaceutics, 12th edition. London: The Pharmaceutical Press, 1994: 760-5.
3. Mulholland P. Displacement values of powder injections. Pharm J 1993; 251: 14-5.
4. Allwood MC, Brown PW. The effect of buffering on the stability of reconstituted benzylpenicillin injection. Int J Pharm Pract 1992; 1: 242-4.
5. Adams P. The stability of reconstituted benzyl penicillin injection in saline when stored in minibags. Pharm J 1992; 249(Suppl): HS20.
6. Allwood MC, Brown PW. The stability of benzylpenicillin injections. Pharm J 1991; 247(Suppl): R12.
7. Stiles ML, Tu Y-H, Allen VA. Stability of cefazolin sodium, cefoxitin sodium, ceftazidime and penicillin G sodium in portable pump reservoirs. Am J Hosp Pharm 1989; 46: 1408-12.
8. Lundgren P, Landersjö L. Studies on the stability and compatibility of drugs in infusion fluids (ii): factors affecting the stability of benzylpenicillin. Acta Pharm Suec 1970; 7: 509-26.

Prepared by

Daniel Murphy and Tim Sizer

Bupivacaine

Approved Name

Bupivacaine hydrochloride

UK Proprietary Name

Marcain (Astra Pharmaceuticals Ltd)

Other Names

—

Product Details

Bupivacaine is available as 10 mL ampoules containing 2.5 mg/mL, 3.75 mg/mL and 5 mg/mL of anhydrous bupivacaine hydrochloride.[1] Injections consist of an isotonic solution of bupivacaine hydrochloride monohydrate. Solutions have a pH of 5.4–5.6 with a specific gravity of 1.004 at 20°C. The sodium content is negligible (0.14 mmol/mL).

Preparation of Injection

The commercially available injections are ready-to-use.

Administration

Bupivacaine is used for local anaesthesia by percutaneous infiltration. It is also used for peripheral nerve block and central nerve block (caudal or epidural). Intravascular administration may cause serious adverse reactions.[1]

Stability in Practice

The manufacturer states that once opened the injection should be used immediately and should be used in an undiluted form. Bupivacaine injections should be stored at 15–30°C and freezing should be avoided.[1]

Infusions should not be used if there is evidence of precipitation or colour change (pink or yellow).

Published Information The chemical stability of bupivacaine 1.25 mg/mL in sodium chloride 0.9% was investigated using HPLC. Samples were stored in polypropylene syringes at 23°C in the light, and 3°C in the dark. Results indicated no detectable loss of bupivacaine after 32 days of storage in the syringes. There was no visible colour changes or evidence of precipitation during the study and no significant changes in pH were observed.[2] *See also* compatibilities.

Incompatibilities The physical stability of 20 mL of bupivacaine (0.25%, 0.5%, and 0.75%) with sodium bicarbonate 4% at volumes of 0.05–0.6 mL has been investigated. Results showed formation of a precipitate within two minutes, and up to two hours with the lowest quantity of sodium bicarbonate.[3,4]

Compatibilities Bupivacaine hydrochloride 7.5 mg/mL has been reported to be visually compatible with hydromorphone hydrochloride 65 mg/mL and morphine sulphate 129 mg/mL when stored in syringes for 30 days at 25°C. Chemical stability was not assessed.[5]

When mixed with iohexol 300 mg/mL, bupivacaine hydrochloride 0.125% and 0.25% has been reported to be visually compatible. No loss of bupivacaine hydrochloride was observed following HPLC analysis after 24 hours storage at room temperature.[6]

Bupivacaine hydrochloride 1.25 mg/mL has been reported to be physically compatible with fentanyl citrate 20 μg/mL when mixed in sodium chloride 0.9%. Little or no loss of either drug was observed after 30 days storage in portable pump reservoirs at 3°C and 23°C.[7]

Solutions of bupivacaine 1 mg/mL and fentanyl citrate 2 μg/mL in sodium chloride 0.9% in PVC bags and polypropylene syringes were reported to be stable for 12 weeks at room temperature and 8°C, in the light.[8]

The stability of solutions containing bupivacaine hydrochloride 625 or 1250 μg/mL in the presence of hydromorphone hydrochloride 20 or 100 μg/mL was investigated by HPLC. The drug combinations were diluted in sodium chloride 0.9% and stored in PVC containers at room temperature (24°C). No significant losses of either drug were recorded over 72 hours.[9]

A similar study of bupivacaine 625 or 1250 μg/mL with morphine sulphate 100 or 500 μg/mL in sodium chloride 0.9% found the combinations to be compatible in fluorescent light at room temperature (23–25°C) in PVC infusion bags for up to 72 hours.[10]

The compatibility and stability of bupivacaine

hydrochloride 2 mg/mL mixed with sufentanil citrate 5 µg/mL has been investigated. Samples were stored in 100 mL PVC portable pump reservoirs for 30 days at 4°C and 32°C. It was concluded that the admixture could be used under patient conditions at 32°C for three days.[11]

The chemical and physical stability of bupivacaine 1.5 mg/mL with fentanyl 10 µg/mL and ketamine 2 mg/mL in sodium chloride 0.9% stored in 5 mL polypropylene syringes was investigated by GC/MS. After storage for one hour at room temperature no significant losses were observed. Similar results were reported for combinations of bupivacaine 1.5 mg/mL, clonidine 30 µg/mL, and morphine 200 µg/mL.[12]

In PVC bags, bupivacaine 1.25 mg/mL was found to be compatible with diamorphine hydrochloride 1.25 µg/mL in sodium chloride 0.9% for 28 days at room temperature in the light. In the same study, bupivacaine 1.25 mg/mL was stable in combination with pethidine 2.5 mg/mL in sodium chloride 0.9% for at least 24 hours at room temperature.[13]

Another study found bupivacaine 1.5 mg/mL with diamorphine 20 µg/mL in sodium chloride 0.9% to be compatible for 20 days at 7°C, 12 days at 25–45°C and six months at -18°C.[14]

Bupivacaine 2.5 and 5 mg/mL stored in PVC bags with diamorphine 0.5, 5, and 10 mg/mL was reported to be stable for eight days at room temperature (25°C) protected from light.[15]

Comments

The limited stability information currently available suggests that bupivacaine hydrochloride solutions diluted in sodium chloride 0.9% to a concentration of 1.25 mg/mL may be stored in polypropylene syringes for at least 28 days at room temperature.

References

1. ABPI. Compendium of data sheets and summaries of product characteristics 1996-1997. London: Datapharm Publications Ltd, 1996: 80-1.
2. Jones JW, Davis AT. Stability of bupivacaine hydrochloride in polypropylene syringes. Am J Hosp Pharm 1993; 50: 2364-5.
3. Bourget P, Bonhomme L, Benhamou D. Factors influencing precipitation of pH-adjusted bupivacaine solutions. J Clin Pharm Ther 1990; 15: 197-204.
4. Trissel LA. Handbook on injectable drugs, 9th edition. Bethesda, MD: American Society of Health-System Pharmacists Inc, 1996: 141-3.
5. Neels JT. Compatibility of bupivacaine hydrochloride with hydromorphone hydrochloride or morphine sulfate. Am J Hosp Pharm 1992; 49: 2149.
6. Van Asten P, et al. Compatibility of bupivacaine and iohexol in two mixtures for paediatric regional anaesthesia. Pharm Weekbl (Sci) 1991; 13: 254-6.
7. Tu Y-H, Stiles ML, Allen LV. Stability of fentanyl citrate and bupivacaine hydrochloride in portable pump reservoirs. Am J Hosp Pharm 1990; 47: 2037-40.
8. Mehta AC, Petty DR. How stable are bupivacaine and fentanyl? Pharm in Pract 1995; 5(1): 21-2.
9. Christen C, Johnson CE, Walters JR. Stability of bupivacaine hydrochloride and hydromorphone hydrochloride during simulated epidural coadministration. Am J Health-Syst Pharm 1996; 53: 170-3.
10. Johnson CE, et al. Compatibility of bupivacaine hydrochloride and morphine sulfate. Am J Health-Syst Pharm 1997; 54: 61-4.
11. Roos PJ, Glerum JH, Schroeders MJH. Effect of glucose 5% solution and bupivacaine hydrochloride on absorption of sufentanil citrate in a portable pump reservoir during storage and simulated infusion by an epidural catheter. Pharm World Sci 1993; 15: 269-75.
12. Christie JM, Jones CW, Markowsky SJ. Chemical compatibility of regional anaesthetic drug combinations. Ann Pharmacother 1992; 26: 1078-80.
13. Grassby PF, Roberts DE. Stability of epidural opiate solutions in 0.9% sodium chloride infusion bags. Int J Pharm Pract 1995; 3: 174-7.
14. Barnes AR, Nash S. Stability of bupivacaine hydrochloride with diamorphine hydrochloride in an epidural infusion. Pharm World Sci 1995; 17: 87-92.
15. Kreeger L, et al. Epidural diamorphine and bupivacaine stability study. Palliative Med 1995; 9: 315-8.

Prepared by

Daniel Murphy and Tim Sizer

Cefotaxime

Approved Name
Cefotaxime

UK Proprietary Name
Claforan (Hoechst Marion Roussel Ltd)

Other Names
Cefacron; Zariviz.

Product Details
Available as glass vials containing the equivalent of 500 mg, 1 g or 2 g of cefotaxime as cefotaxime sodium. The 1 g vials are available in packs of 50 for hospital pharmacy use only.[1]

The injection consists of a sterile white to slightly creamy coloured freeze-dried powder of cefotaxime sodium. Approximately 1.05 g of cefotaxime sodium is equivalent to 1 g of cefotaxime. Each gram of cefotaxime sodium contains 2.09 mmol of sodium.

Displacement values are: 0.2 mL/500 mg, 0.5 mL/1 g, and 1.2 mL/2 g. A cefotaxime 10% solution reconstituted with water for injection has a pH of approximately 5.5.

Preparation of Injection
The content of each vial may be reconstituted by the addition of water for injection to form a straw coloured solution (*see* table).

Variations in the intensity of the colour of the freshly prepared solution does not indicate change in potency or safety, provided the recommended storage conditions are observed.

Solutions may be further diluted in the following diluents: compound sodium lactate; glucose 5%; glucose 10%; glucose 5% and sodium chloride 0.2%; glucose 5% and sodium chloride 0.45%; glucose 5% and sodium chloride 0.9%; invert sugar injection; sodium chloride 0.9%; sodium lactate M/6; and water for injection.

Administration
Cefotaxime may be administered by intravenous bolus injection over 3–5 minutes, or by infusion in 40–100 mL of fluid over 20–60 minutes. Cefotaxime may also be administered by deep intramuscular injection.

Approximately 50–80% of an intravenous cefotaxime dose is excreted unchanged in the urine within 24 hours of injection. Cefotaxime is metabolised, in the liver, primarily to desacetylcefotaxime. Two other inactive metabolites have also been identified. The desacetyl metabolite exhibits antimicrobial activity, but less than that of cefotaxime itself, and has a half-life of about 1.5 hours, i.e. longer than cefotaxime which is about one hour. The desacetyl metabolite has a similar acute toxicity profile to the parent molecule.[2]

The total body clearance of cefotaxime has been reduced in patients with normal and reduced renal function by the concomitant administration of azlocillin or mezlocillin. Probenicid competes for renal tubular secretion with cefotaxime resulting in higher and prolonged plasma concentrations of cefotaxime and its desacetyl metabolite.

Stability in Practice
The primary factor in determining the stability of cefotaxime sodium in aqueous solution is solution pH. Cefotaxime is most stable at pH 4.3–6.2.[3] At low pH, beta-lactam ring hydrolysis (lactonisation) occurs most readily, while amide side chain hydrolysis predominates at higher pH values.[3]

Cefotaxime stability is also affected by light and temperature, with solutions most stable when refrigerated.[4,5]

In the UK, the manufacturer states that it is preferable to use freshly prepared cefotaxime solutions. However, if this is not possible, reconstituted solutions are said to be stable for 24 hours when stored in a refrigerator.

Published Information   Although it is preferable to use only freshly reconstituted solutions for both intravenous and intramuscular administration, cefotaxime reconstituted with water for injection has been reported to be stable for 24 hours at room temperature (at or below 22°C), for ten days when refrigerated (below 5°C), and for at least 13 weeks when frozen.[6]

Frozen cefotaxime solutions should be thawed at room temperature before use. The reconstituted solution is subsequently stable for 24 hours at room

Vial size (g)	Amount of water for injection to be added (mL)	Approximate available volume (mL)	Approximate concentration (mg/mL)
0.5	2	2.2	227
1.0	4	4.5	222
2.0	10	11.2	179

temperature and for ten days when refrigerated. Any unused solutions of frozen material should be discarded. Solutions of cefotaxime should not be refrozen.[6]

Solutions of cefotaxime in glucose 5% or sodium chloride 0.9% stored in PVC containers and disposable glass or plastic syringes were stable for 24 hours at room temperature (at or below 22°C), for five days in a refrigerator (at or below 5°C), and for 13 weeks when frozen.[6]

Cefotaxime 2 mg/mL in 1 mL polypropylene syringes retained its potency for at least seven days in a refrigerator (4–8°C) as assessed by a biological assay.[7]

The chemical stability of cefotaxime sodium 1 mg/1 mL in water for injection was investigated at a range of pH values. Samples were stored in 60 mL amber glass bottles at 24°C, 4°C, and -10°C and analysed by HPLC. Additionally, the stability of cefotaxime sodium 10 mg/mL in glucose 5% and sodium chloride 0.9% in PVC bags at the same storage temperatures was investigated. Results indicated that decomposition was first-order, the optimum pH range for stability being pH 4.3–6.2. All samples were stable for 24 hours at 24°C, 22 days at 4°C, and 16 weeks at -10°C. There was a negligible change in pH.[3]

The chemical stability of cefotaxime sodium 10 mg/mL was investigated in sodium chloride 0.9% minibags, in ready-to-use metronidazole minibags, and in sodium chloride 0.9% minibags with metronidazole hydrochloride 500 mg added. Analysis was by stability indicating HPLC assay. All minibags were made of PVC and were stored at 5°C and 28°C. Results indicated that cefotaxime was stable for 96 hours at 5°C in the presence of reconstituted or ready-to-use metronidazole, for 24 hours at 28°C in the presence of reconstituted metronidazole, and for 19 hours at 28°C in the presence of ready-to-use metronidazole.[8]

The chemical stability of cefotaxime sodium 10 mg/mL was investigated in ready-to-use glass bottles of metronidazole 500 mg/100 mL. The cefotaxime was reconstituted with 5 mL of sodium chloride 0.9%. Analysis was by HPLC. Results indicated that cefotaxime was stable for 72 hours at 8°C in ready-to-use metronidazole injection.[9]

Unpublished Information The chemical stability of cefotaxime sodium 1 g/4 mL or 2 g/10 mL in water for injection stored in 5 mL polypropylene syringes stoppered with high density polyethylene plugs was investigated by HPLC and microbiological assay. Samples were stored at 4°C and 25°C in the light. Results indicated that solutions stored at 4°C were stable for seven days, while those stored at 25°C were stable for 24 hours.[10]

The chemical stability of cefotaxime sodium 500 mg/50 mL in sodium chloride 0.9% stored in PVC minibags at room temperature and in a refrigerator (2–8°C) was investigated by HPLC. Results indicated that solutions stored at room temperature were stable for 24 hours while those stored in a refrigerator were stable for ten days.[11]

A similar study of cefotaxime sodium 1 g/50 mL in sodium chloride 0.9% stored in minibags at room temperature and in a refrigerator (2–8°C) indicated that solutions stored at room temperature were stable for 24 hours while those stored in a refrigerator were stable for ten days.[11]

Incompatibilities Cefotaxime is reported to be chemically or physically incompatible with the following drug substances: alkaline solutions; allopurinol sodium; aminophylline; doxapram; filgrastim; fluconazole; hetastarch; and vancomycin.[12]

Compatibilities The manufacturer states that cefotaxime should not be mixed with other antibiotics in the same syringe or infusion. However, cefotaxime is reported to be stable for at least 72 hours when refrigerated in lignocaine 1%. Cefotaxime is also reported to be stable for 24 hours in a refrigerator when mixed with metronidazole 500 mg/100 mL.[8,9]

Cefotaxime is reported to be stable for at least 24 hours when stored at room temperature in peritoneal dialysis fluid containing heparin 500 units/L or insulin 20 units/L.[1]

Comments

Cefotaxime in aqueous injections exhibits reasonable stability when refrigerated at pH 4.3–6.2; at least five days at 4°C and 24 hours at room temperature.

References

1. ABPI. Compendium of data sheets and summaries of product characteristics 1996-1997. London: Datapharm Publications Ltd, 1996: 934-5.
2. Doerr BL, et al. Cefotaxime toxicity studies: a review of pre-clinical studies and some clinical reports. Rev Infect Dis 1982; 4(Suppl): S354-9.
3. Das Gupta V. Stability of cefotaxime sodium as determined by high-performance liquid chromatography. J Pharm Sci 1984; 73: 565-7.
4. Vilanova B, et al. Alkaline hydrolysis of cefotaxime: A HPLC and ^{1}H NMR study. J Pharm Sci 1994; 83: 322-7.
5. Lerner DA, et al. Photodegradation paths of cefotaxime. J Pharm Sci 1988; 77: 699-703.
6. Physicians desk reference 1997. Montvale, NJ: Medical Economics Company Inc, 1997: 1259-61.
7. Ahmed ST, Parkinson R. The stability of drugs in prefilled syringes. Hosp Pharm Pract 1992; 2: 285-9.
8. Belliveau PP, Nightingale CH, Quintiliani R. Stability of cefotaxime sodium and metronidazole in 0.9% sodium chloride injection or in ready-to-use metronidazole bags. Am J Hosp Pharm 1995; 52: 1561-3.
9. Rivers TE, McBride HA, Trang JM. Stability of cefotaxime sodium and metronidazole in an IV admixture at 8°C. Am J Hosp Pharm 1991; 48: 2638-40.
10. Owen D. Personal communication, 1994.
11. Wicker S. Personal communication, 1994.
12. Trissel LA. Handbook on injectable Drugs, 9th edition. Bethesda, MD: American Society of Health-System Pharmacists Inc, 1996: 192-6.

Prepared by

Brian Baker and Christine Trehane

Ceftazidime

Approved Name
Ceftazidime

UK Proprietary Name
Fortum (Glaxo Wellcome)
Kefadim (Eli Lilly)

Other Names
Ceptaz; Fortaz; Tazidime; Tazicef.

Product Details
In the UK, ceftazidime is available, for intramuscular or intravenous injection, in glass vials containing the equivalent of 250 mg (Fortum only), 500 mg, 1 g, 2 g or 3 g (Fortum only) of ceftazidime as the pentahydrate.[1,2] Glass vials containing ceftazidime 2 g for intravenous infusion are also commercially available. Fortum Saline Infusion kit containing ceftazidime 2 g, 50 mL of sodium chloride 0.9% intravenous infusion and the disposables required to prepare the kit are also available. Other pack sizes are available in other countries.[3]

The commercially available injections consist of a sterile white powder of ceftazidime pentahydrate with 118 mg of sodium carbonate per gram of ceftazidime. Each gram of ceftazidime contains approximately 54 mg (2.3 mmol) of sodium. All sizes of Fortum vials are supplied under reduced pressure and Kefadim vials may contain a vacuum. As the product dissolves, the sodium salt of the ceftazidime is produced, carbon dioxide is released, and a positive pressure develops.

The Ceptaz dosage form contains 349 mg of L-arginine per gram of ceftazidime instead of sodium carbonate and it dissolves without gas evolution.

Preparation of Injection
The content of each vial is reconstituted with the required volume of diluent to form a solution varying in colour from pale straw to amber, depending on the diluent and concentration. The volumes for reconstitution recommended by the manufacturers are shown in the table opposite.

The displacement value for Kefadim is 0.6 mL/g. The displacement value for Fortum varies with vial size: 0.2 mL/250 mg; 0.45 mL/500 mg; 0.9 mL/1 g; 1.8 mL/2 g; and 2.7 mL/3 g.

The manufacturers state that the following injections are suitable for the reconstitution of ceftazidime at concentrations between 1 mg/mL and 40 mg/mL: compound sodium lactate; dextran 40 10% in glucose 5%; dextran 40 10% in sodium chloride 0.9%; dextran 70 6% in glucose 5%; dextran 70 6% in sodium chloride 0.9%; glucose 5%; glucose 10%; sodium chloride 0.18% and glucose 4%; sodium chloride 0.225% and glucose 5%; sodium chloride 0.45% and glucose 5%; sodium chloride 0.9%; sodium chloride 0.9% and glucose 5%; sodium lactate M/6; and water for injection.

Ceftazidime is less stable in sodium bicarbonate than in other intravenous fluids and this is not recommended as a diluent.

The pH of the reconstituted solution depends on the solvent used. The manufacturers state that reconstituted Kefadim has a pH of 5–7.5 and reconstituted Fortum a pH between 6–8.

Administration
Ceftazidime may be administered as an intravenous bolus injection, in a suitable diluent, over 3–5 minutes. It may also be administered as an intravenous infusion over 15–30 minutes.

Before administration, any carbon dioxide bubbles produced during reconstitution should be expelled from the syringe or infusion container; alternatively the infusion should be stopped before the gas is infused.

Ceftazidime is not metabolised and 90–96% of a dose is excreted by renal elimination. Biliary excretion accounts for less than 1% of a dose.

Stability in Practice
In the UK, the manufacturers state that it is preferable to use freshly reconstituted ceftazidime solutions. However, potency is retained when solutions are stored refrigerated for 24 hours.

Variations in the intensity of the colour of freshly prepared solutions does not affect potency, provided they are prepared and stored within the manufacturers stated recommendations.

The degradation of ceftazidime in aqueous solu-

Vial size	Route of administration	Amount of diluent to be added (mL)	Approximate available volume (mL)	Approximate concentration (mg/mL)
250 mg (Fortum)	IM	1.0	1.2	210
250 mg (Fortum)	IV	2.5	2.7	90
500 mg (Fortum)	IM	1.5	1.95	260
500 mg (Kefadim)	IM	1.5	1.8	280
500 mg (Fortum)	IV	5.0	5.45	90
500 mg (Kefadim)	IV	5.0	5.3	100
1 g (Fortum)	IM	3.0	3.9	260
1g (Kefadim)	IM	3.0	3.6	280
1g (Fortum)	IV	10.0	10.9	90
1g (Kefadim)	IV	10.0	10.6	100
2g (Fortum)	IV bolus	10.0	11.8	170
2g (Kefadim)	IV bolus	10.0	11.2	180
2g (Fortum)*	IV infusion	50.0	51.8	40
2g (Kefadim)	IV infusion	100.0	100	20
3g (Fortum)	IV bolus	15.0	17.7	170
3g (Fortum)*†	IV infusion	75.0	77.7	40

* Water for injection should not be used to reconstitute these strengths as hypotonic solutions are formed.

† The solvent needs to be added in two stages with the gas pressure released between the two stages.

tion is a complex process and is reported to be first-order. The reaction initially involves loss of pyridine and opening of the beta-lactam ring. Further inter- and intra-molecular reactions then occur leading to a complex mixture of degradation products. The degradation products have not been fully characterised or subjected to specific toxicity testing.[4]

Published Information The microbiological stability of ceftazidime 100 mg/mL (with sodium carbonate) was investigated in water for injection in syringes made up of a polypropylene barrel and polyethylene plunger sealed with a multi-add syringe cap. Bio-assay was performed according to the biological assay for antibiotics method A of the *British Pharmacopoeia 1988*, using *Pseudomonas aeruginosa* NCTC 8626 as the test organism. Storage was between 4–8°C for up to 14 days, details of light protection were not indicated. It was postulated that

the smaller the volume the greater the potential for interaction with syringe material or atmospheric oxygen due to a higher surface volume ratio. Therefore, in the study the smallest volume likely to be delivered from these syringes to patients, i.e. 0.4 mL, was tested. Results showed that ceftazidime retained its potency against the test organism over the test period of 14 days, although a low result of 87% was obtained at day seven; this appeared to have risen again by day nine. Within the first seven days the solutions had become a dark yellow colour.[5]

The chemical stability of ceftazidime (containing sodium carbonate) was investigated in sterile water for injection stored in polypropylene syringes and in the original bulk glass containers. Analysis was by a modified stability indicating HPLC assay. The drug concentrations were 100 mg/mL and 200 mg/mL. Storage was at one of the following six temperature combinations: (i) ambient temperature (21–23°C) for up to eight hours; (ii) 4°C for up to 96 hours; (iii) -20°C for 28 days and then 21–23°C for up to eight hours; (iv) -20°C for 28 days and then 4°C for up to 96 hours; (v) -20°C for 91 days and then 21–23°C for up to eight hours; (vi) -20°C for 91 days and then 4°C for up to 96 hours.[6]

All solutions were stable over the entire study period. When the drug was stored under conditions (i) and (ii) the ceftazidime concentrations remained above 95% of the initial values in either container for the entire study period. When the drug was frozen for 28 days then subsequently stored under conditions (iii) or (iv), ceftazidime concentrations remained above 93% in either container for the study period. When the drug was frozen for 91 days then subsequently stored under conditions (v) or (vi), the ceftazidime concentrations only marginally met the stability criteria. Accuracy, or percentage of error, of the method was calculated to be 3–5%. There were no colour or other visual changes in any of the samples at any point in the study.

A separate set of ceftazidime vials were reconstituted with sterile water for injection and stored under the same conditions for particle analysis, using the method specified in the *United States Pharmacopeia* volume XXI (USP). Particle counts for each storage condition and for each concentration were well within the USP recommendations.[6]

The chemical stability of ceftazidime with arginine was investigated in sterile water for injection in polypropylene syringes. Analysis was by stability indicating HPLC. The drug concentration was 100 mg/mL. Storage conditions were as follows: (i) 22°C for 24 hours; (ii) 4°C for seven days followed by 22°C for 24 hours; (iii) 4°C for ten days followed by 22°C for 24 hours; (iv) -20°C for 91 days followed by 22°C for 24 hours; (v) -20°C for 91 days followed by 4°C for seven days followed by 22°C for 24 hours. Syringes were protected from light.

Results showed that ceftazidime concentrations in all samples remained greater than 90% during the entire study. No peaks for degradation products were noted. The colour of the solutions changed to dark yellow during storage, but no precipitate was detected. Mean pH values for all the solutions dropped from, pH 6.54–6.65 to 6.10–6.17 at the end of the study.[7] This study suggested that ceftazidime with arginine may be preferable to ceftazidime with sodium carbonate when solutions are stored in

syringes or infusion pump reservoirs as the gas bubbles produced by the latter formulation may make it difficult to handle.

The stability of ceftazidime 1 g (with sodium carbonate) was investigated in 50 mL minibags of sodium chloride 0.9%. Analysis was by stability indicating HPLC assay. Storage was at -20°C for up to 97 days. Samples were thawed in a fan assisted oven set at 30°C for 45 minutes which raised the temperature of the minibags to 15°C. Samples were then refrigerated at 5°C for four days, then left at room temperature for a further 24 hours.

In addition, a microbiological diffusion assay was carried out using a spore suspension of *Bacillus subtilis* 1904 E as the assay organism and Oxoid antibiotic agar No.2 with the addition of sodium citrate 0.3% as the growth medium. Standard ceftazidime solution was diluted to 5 mg/mL, 2.5 mg/mL, and 1.25 mg/L and test samples were diluted, with buffer, to give approximately the same concentrations. The plates were incubated at 37°C for 18 hours and the diameter of the inhibition zones measured.

The results showed good agreement between the two analytical methods. The potency loss was initially rapid with a 3.3% drop in the first 16 days, but then slowed with a further 3.5% drop in the next 81 days. The drop in potency is more rapid during refrigeration and room temperature storage than during frozen storage. After 29 days frozen storage followed by four days refrigeration and 24 hours room temperature storage the concentration was 92.2% of the original, but following 69 days frozen storage followed by the same refrigerated and room temperature storage, the HPLC results indicated more than 10% degradation.[8]

The chemical stability of ceftazidime 1 g (with sodium carbonate) reconstituted according to the manufacturer's instructions then transferred to 50 mL minibags of sodium chloride 0.9% was investigated. Analysis was by stability indicating HPLC assay. The results showed that ceftazidime concentration remained above 90% for 20 days, but was less than 90% at 28 days when stored at 5°C.[9]

Unpublished Information The chemical stability of ceftazidime 100 mg/mL in water for injections has been investigated stored in polypropylene syringes. Analysis was by HPLC, with samples stored at 6°C, 22°C, and 40°C for up to seven days. Results suggested that ceftazidime was stable for up to five days in polypropylene syringes at 6°C.

The chemical stability of ceftazidime 20 mg/mL was investigated in sodium chloride 0.9% in 100 mL PVC minibags. Analysis was by HPLC assay with samples stored at 2–6°C for 60 days. Results suggested that samples were stable for up to 14 days.[10]

The stability of ceftazidime 2 g in sodium chloride 0.9% 50 mL minibags and in 100 mL of sodium chloride 0.9% in a glass infusion bottle was determined by HPLC assay. Storage was at 4–8°C in a refrigerator and at -30°C in a freezer for the minibags. The infusion bottle was stored only in the refrigerator. Results suggested that ceftazidime was stable for seven days in both the minibags and infusion bottle at 4–8°C. The minibags, when defrosted, after one month, were stable for a further seven days at 4–8°C.[11]

Incompatibilities Ceftazidime is reported to be incompatible with: aminoglycosides; amsacrine; fluconazole; idarubicin; ranitidine; and vancomycin.

Compatibilities Ceftazidime is not normally mixed with other active ingredients, however, at a concentration of 4 mg/mL, it has been found to be compatible for 24 hours at room temperature in sodium chloride 0.9% when mixed with cefuroxime sodium 3 mg/mL; and heparin 10 µg/mL or 50 µg/mL. Ceftazidime (Kefadim) is also reported to be stable with the above combinations in glucose 5%. Additionally, ceftazidime (Fortum) has been tested with hydrocortisone sodium phosphate 1 mg/mL in sodium chloride 0.9% or glucose 5% and cloxacillin (as the sodium salt) 4 mg/mL in sodium chloride 0.9% and been found to be stable for the same length of time under the same conditions.[1,2]

Ceftazidime has been reported to be compatible with metronidazole. The chemical stability of ceftazidime 1 g (with sodium carbonate) was investigated, reconstituted with sodium chloride 0.9% to a concentration of 200 mg/mL, then added to PVC bags of ready-to-use metronidazole 5 mg/mL injection, to a final volume of approximately 105 mL. Analysis was by stability indicating HPLC assay for both the ceftazidime and metronidazole. Samples were stored at 8°C for up to 72 hours, details of light protection were not indicated. Results indicated that the percentage of the initial concentration remaining at all times for ceftazidime was 96.9–100.8% and for metronidazole was 96.5–105.8%. None of the samples showed any signs of colour change or precipitation.[12]

Comments
—

References

1. ABPI. Compendium of data sheets and summaries of product characteristics 1996-1997. London: Datapharm Publications Ltd, 1996: 393-5.
2. ABPI. Compendium of data sheets and summaries of product characteristics 1996-1997. London: Datapharm Publications Ltd, 1996: 529-30.
3. Trissel LA. Handbook on injectable drugs, 9th edition. Bethesda, MD: American Society of Health-System Pharmacists Inc, 1996: 206-12.
4. Dick F. Personal communication, 1997.
5. Ahmed ST, Parkinson R. The stability of drugs in pre-filled syringes: flucloxacillin, ampicillin, cefuroxime, cefotaxime and ceftazidime. Hosp Pharm Pract 1992; 2: 285-9.
6. Stewart JT, et al. Stability of ceftazidime in plastic syringes and glass vials under various storage conditions. Am J Hosp Pharm 1992; 49: 2765-8.
7. Nahata MC, Morosco RS, Fox JL. Stability of ceftazidime (with arginine) stored in plastic syringes at three temperatures. Am J Hosp Pharm 1992; 49: 2954-6.
8. Brown AF, Harvey, DA, Hoddinott DJ. Freeze thaw stability of ceftazidime. Br J Parenter Ther 1985; 6(2): 43, 45, 50.
9. Brown AF, Harvey DA, Hoddinott DJ, Britton KJ. Freeze-thaw stability of antibiotics used in an IV additive service. Br J Parenter Ther 1986; 7(2): 42–4.
10. Allwood MC. Personal communication, 1996.
11. Whicker, S. Personal communication, 1996.
12. Rivers TE, Webster AA. Stability of ceftizoxime sodium, ceftriaxone sodium and ceftazidime with metronidazole in ready-to-use metronidazole bags. Am J Health-Syst Pharm 1995; 52: 2568-70.

Prepared by

Christine Trehane

Cefuroxime

Approved Name

Cefuroxime sodium

UK Proprietary Name

Zinacef (Glaxo Wellcome)

Other Names

—

Product Details

Glass vials containing a white to faintly yellow coloured powder of 250mg, 750mg, or 1.5g of cefuroxime as the sodium salt. The vials have a pH of 6–8.5 when reconstituted. Sodium content is 1.8 mmol/750mg. Frozen premixed solutions have a pH of 5–7.5.[1]

Two infusion kits are also available containing a cefuroxime 750mg vial and a sodium chloride 0.9% 50mL infusion bag in one kit, and a cefuroxime 750mg vial and metronidazole 0.5% 100mL infusion bag in the other.

Preparation of Injection

Cefuroxime 250mg should be reconstituted with at least 2mL of water for injection, cefuroxime 750mg with at least 6mL of water for injection, and cefuroxime 1.5g with 15mL of water for injection.

If more accurate reconstitution is required (e.g. for paediatric use) the displacement value is 0.18mL/250mg.[2]

If using the infusion kits, a transfer needle is used to reconstitute the vial with the infusion solution.

Administration

Cefuroxime may be administered by slow intravenous injection over 3–5 minutes, or by intermittent infusion of up to 30 minutes duration in compound sodium lactate, glucose 4% with sodium chloride 0.18%, glucose 5%, metronidazole 0.5%, or sodium chloride 0.9%.[3]

A suspension of cefuroxime 250mg/mL or 750mg/3mL, in water for injection, may also be administered by intramuscular injection.[3]

Stability in Practice

The optimum range for cefuroxime stability is pH 4.5–7.3.[4] Cefuroxime is thermolabile and rapidly degrades at room temperature. Solutions should be protected from light.

Published Information   Cefuroxime has been reported to be stable at concentrations of 750mg and 1.5g in 50mL PVC minibags of sodium chloride 0.9% and glucose 5% stored for 20 days at 4°C.[5] Cefuroxime 250mg/2mL has been reported to be stable for at least seven days in 1mL syringes, although changes in the colour of the solution were noted.[6]

Cefuroxime 1.5g in 50mL sodium chloride 0.9% minibags is said to have a shelf-life of 19 days at 7°C and 24 hours at room temperature. Cefuroxime 1.5g in 50mL glucose 5% minibags is said to have a shelf-life of 20 days at 4°C and 24 hours at room temperature.[7]

Unpublished Information   Cefuroxime 75mg/mL stored in syringes is said to lose approximately 5% of cefuroxime after 12 days. Thus, a shelf-life of 12 days has been assigned to this product if stored at, or below, 5°C.[8]

Cefuroxime 750mg in 50mL glucose 5% is said to be stable for 180 days at -20°C followed by seven days at 5°C.[9]

Studies into the long-term stability of cefuroxime 750mg/50mL in polypropylene syringes have shown less than 10% loss of cefuroxime over five years at -20°C, although a significant increase in yellow colouration was observed.[10]

The stability of cefuroxime 750mg in metronidazole 5mg/mL solution stored frozen in 100mL bags has been investigated. No loss or breakdown of either drug was said to have occurred after six months. Once thawed, it is recommended that bags are used within three days. A precipitation, probably metronidazole, occurs but disappears once the solution reaches room temperature.[11]

Incompatibilities   Cefuroxime has been reported to be physically or chemically incompatible with the following drug substances: aminoglycosides; clarithromycin; filgrastim; fluconazole; and vinorelbine.[1,3,12]

Compatibilities   Cefuroxime 750mg and 1.5g admixtures in 100 mL of metronidazole 0.5% infusion are stable for seven days.[13,14]

Cefuroxime stability in glucose 5% or sodium chloride 0.9% is not affected by the presence of hydrocortisone sodium phosphate.[3]

Cefuroxime is compatible with aqueous solutions of lignocaine hydrochloride 1%.[3]

Comments

When frozen at -20°C, cefuroxime sodium shows good stability with shelf-lives of more than six months reported. When refrigerated, some degradation occurs, with up to 10% loss of cefuroxime within three weeks. Degradation is more rapid at room temperature and the reconstituted injection should be used within 24 hours.

References

1. Trissel LA. Handbook on injectable drugs, 9th edition. Bethesda, MD: American Society of Health-System Pharmacists Inc, 1996: 220-4.
2. Mulholland P. Displacement values of powder injections. Pharm J 1993; 251: 14-5.
3. ABPI. Compendium of data sheets and summaries of product characteristics 1996-1997. London: Datapharm Publications Ltd, 1996: 402-4.
4. Das Gupta V, Stewart KR. Stability of cefuroxime sodium in some aqueous buffered solutions and intravenous admixtures. J Clin Hosp Pharm 1986; 11: 47-54.
5. Small D. The stability of cefuroxime in infusion solutions. Pharm J 1992; 248(Suppl): HS40.
6. Ahmed ST, Parkinson R. The stability of drugs in pre-filled syringes: flucloxacillin, ampicillin, cefuroxime, cefotaxime and ceftazidime. Hosp Pharm Pract 1992; 2: 285-9.
7. Coomber PA, Jefferies JP, Woodford JD. High-performance liquid chromatographic determination of cefuroxime. Analyst 1982; 107: 1451-6.
8. Allwood MC. Personal communication, 1996.
9. Baxter Healthcare Ltd. Personal communication, 1995.
10. Chandarana N. Personal communication, 1997.
11. Midcalf B. Personal communication, 1996.
12. Taylor A. A physical compatibility study of clarithromycin injection with other commonly used injectable drugs. Pharm in Pract 1997; 7(9): 473-6.
13. Barnes AR. Chemical stabilities of cefuroxime sodium and metronidazole in an admixture for intravenous infusion. J Clin Pharm Ther 1990; 15: 187-96.
14. McLaughlin JP, Simpson C, Taylor RA. How stable are Zinacef and Metrovex: the stability of cefuroxime sodium and metronidazole infusion when stored in a refrigerator. Pharm in Pract 1995; 5(3): 100-6.

Prepared by

Christine Clarke

Cephradine

Approved Name
Cephradine

UK Proprietary Name
Velosef (Bristol-Myers Squibb)

Other Names
Cefradine.

Product Details
Available as vials containing the equivalent of 500 mg and 1 g of cephradine as a sterile powder blend with L-arginine.[1] When reconstituted with water for injection, the resulting solution has a pH of 8.5–9.5. An aqueous solution containing 50 mg/mL of cephradine is approximately isotonic.[1]

Cephradine injection (arginine blend) is sodium free.

Preparation of Injection
For intramuscular administration, cephradine should be reconstituted with either sodium chloride 0.9% or water for injection. For the 500 mg vial, 2 mL of diluent should be used; 4 mL of diluent should be used for the 1 g vial.

For intravenous injection, solutions should be prepared by adding 5 mL of diluent to the 500 mg vial or 10 mL of diluent to the 1 g vial. Suitable diluents are glucose 5%, sodium chloride 0.9%, and water for injection. If more accurate reconstitution is required (e.g. for paediatric use) the following powder displacement value may be used: 0.4 mL/500 mg.[2]

Reconstituted injections may vary in colour from light to straw yellow. However, this does not indicate any loss of potency.[1]

For continuous or intermittent infusion, suitable infusion fluids are: compound sodium lactate; glucose 5%; glucose 10%; glucose 5% in compound sodium lactate; glucose 5% in Ringer's solution; Ringer's solution; sodium chloride 0.9%; and water for injection. Note that only cephradine solubilised with arginine may be reconstituted with solutions containing calcium salts, such as Ringer's solution.

Administration
Cephradine may be administered by intramuscular injection, intravenous injection over 3–5 minutes, or by continuous intravenous infusion.

Stability in Practice
The major degradation route of cephradine is thought to be the opening of the beta-lactam ring by hydrolysis.[3]

The stability of cephradine solutions is concentration and temperature dependent. It is recommended that solutions intended for intramuscular and intravenous injection should be used within two hours if kept at room temperature, and within 12 hours if stored in a refrigerator at 5°C.[1]

Infusions are reported to be stable for 24 hours at room temperature or seven days at 5°C at concentrations up to 10 mg/mL, and for ten hours at room temperature or 48 hours at 5°C at concentrations up to 50 mg/mL.[1]

Cephradine solutions should be protected from strong light or direct sunlight. Vials should be stored at room temperature.

Published Information The stability of cephradine 100 mg/mL aqueous solutions stored at -20°C, 4°C, and room temperature for six weeks was investigated using an HPLC assay.[3] No degradation of cephradine over this period was observed in samples stored at -20°C. However, samples stored at 4°C showed some deterioration in potency, with 10% decomposition after 24 hours storage. Samples stored at room temperature deteriorated more rapidly, with greater than 10% decomposition becoming apparent after two hours. Light appeared to have no significant effect on stability with degradation occurring, it was suggested, as a result of hydrolysis of the beta-lactam ring.

The stability of cephradine 500 mg in 100 mL of sodium chloride 0.9%, stored for seven days in the dark, in a refrigerator and at room temperature (20°C) in minibags was investigated using a stability indicating HPLC assay.[4] Prolonged storage at room temperature showed two major breakdown products. Based on a 10% loss in potency, it was concluded that the infusion was stable for seven days in a refrigerator, but only two days at room temperature (20°C).

The stability of cephradine in plastic syringes was investigated by reconstituting 1 g of cephradine with 10 mL of water for injection which was then stored in a polypropylene syringe in a refrigerator (6°C).[5] Samples were withdrawn at intervals over two days and analysed using an HPLC assay. The solution degraded according to first-order kinetics, with 5% loss of cephradine after 5.7 hours, and 10% loss after 11.9 hours. Evidence of sorption to the syringe nozzle was also noted. It was therefore concluded that a maximum shelf-life of 12 hours was appropriate for the sample.

A cephradine-arginine 1% solution was found to be more stable than a cephradine-sodium carbonate 1% solution in several intravenous fluids. However, this finding was only significant at low concentrations since at cephradine 5% and cephradine 25% concentrations differences in stability between the two formulations were not substantial.[6]

Incompatibilities Cephradine (sodium carbonate blend) is incompatible with solutions containing calcium salts. The arginine blend has not been reported to exhibit the same reactions.

Ascorbic acid, carbenicillin, kanamycin, methicillin, and vitamin B complex, have been reported to degrade at a faster than expected rate in cephradine-sodium carbonate solutions.[7]

Compatibilities Procaine hydrochloride 2% solution has been used to reconstitute cephradine injection (sodium carbonate formulation) for intramuscular injection. Studies in 16 subjects showed that the bioavailability of cephradine from this admixture was not significantly different when compared to similar injections reconstituted with sterile water.[8]

Comments

Once reconstituted the stability of cephradine injection is concentration and temperature dependent. Published information is limited and should be interpreted with care. In common clinical practice, solutions containing cephradine 10 mg/mL should be used within 24 hours at room temperature or within seven days if refrigerated. A more concentrated solution of cephradine 50 mg/mL will remain stable for ten hours at room temperature or 48 hours at 5°C.

References

1. ABPI. Compendium of data sheets and summaries of product characteristics 1996-1997. London: Datapharm Publications Ltd, 1996: 1146-7.
2. Mulholland P. Displacement values of powder injections. Pharm J 1993; 251: 14-5.
3. Mehta AC, McCarthy M, Calvert RT. The chemical stability of cephradine injection solutions. Intensive Therapy Clin Monit 1988; 9: 195-6.
4. Adams P. The stability of reconstituted cephradine injection in 0.9 per cent sodium chloride when stored in minibags. Pharm J 1992; 249(Suppl): HS20.
5. Grassby PF. The stability of cephradine injections in polypropylene syringes. Pharm J 1992; 248(Suppl): HS25.
6. Wang YJ, Monkhouse DC. Soluuion stability of cephradine neutralised with arginine or sodium bicarbonate. Am J Hosp Pharm 1983; 40: 432-4.
7. Bristol-Myers Squibb. Personal communication, 1997.
8. Vukovich RA, Sugerman AA, Fields LA. Effect of 2% procaine hydrochloride solution on the bioavailability of cephradine after intramuscular injection. Curr Ther Res 1975; 18: 711-9.

Prepared by

Denise Fenton

Ciprofloxacin

Approved Name
Ciprofloxacin lactate

UK Proprietary Name
Ciproxin (Bayer plc)

Other Names
—

Product Details
Glass bottles containing a clear, almost colourless to pale yellow solution with the equivalent of 100mg, 200mg or 400mg ciprofloxacin (as the lactate) in sodium chloride 0.9%. The injection is also available in PVC minibags containing 200mg or 400mg of ciprofloxacin in 100mL or 200mL of sodium chloride 0.9%.

Ciprofloxacin lactate 127mg is equivalent to ciprofloxacin 100mg. The infusion solution contains sodium chloride 0.9% and lactic acid 0.01%. The sodium content of the injection solution is approximately 1.54mmol/mL. The injection has a pH of 3.9–4.5.[1-3]

Preparation of Injection
The infusion is supplied ready-to-use, but may be further diluted in fructose 10%, glucose 5%, glucose 10%, Ringer's solution, sodium chloride 0.9%, or solutions of glucose and sodium chloride.[1]

Administration
Ciprofloxacin injection may be infused directly into a large vein, over a period of 30–60 minutes. Longer infusion periods may be used but are not recommended as ciprofloxacin injections are sensitive to sunlight and UV light.

Stability in Practice
Ciprofloxacin is a synthetic 4-quinolone derivative with generally good aqueous stability. Ciprofloxacin lactate has optimum stability in the range pH 3.9–4.5. Solubility decreases markedly when the pH approaches its isoelectric point (pH 7.4).

If refrigerated, crystals may form which will re-dissolve at room temperature, without significantly affecting the characteristics of the injection. Solutions should not be infused if turbidity or crystals are observed. Exposure to temperatures above 40°C should be avoided.[1,4]

Ciprofloxacin will degrade in solution to 7-(2 aminoethylamino)-1-cycloproyl-6-fluoro 1,4-oxo-3-quinoline carboxylic acid.[5] Ciprofloxacin is also prone to chelation with divalent and trivalent cations, which may result in precipitation.[6]

Loss of ciprofloxacin may occur in PVC containers due to absorption or sorption.[6] Although no drug loss due to sorption was detected by HPLC when a solution of ciprofloxacin 0.8mg/mL in PVC bags was run though infusion sets at about 4mL/min.[7] Solutions may also cause the leaching of small amounts of plasticizer from PVC containers (e.g. DEHP and BEHP).[6]

Ciprofloxacin is sensitive to UV light, losing potency if exposed to UVA at a wavelength of 320–400nm. The bi-products of photodegradation are reported to be toxic, and may induce photosensitivity in some patients, although the phototoxicity of ciprofloxacin is reputedly the least of the commercially available fluoroquinolones.[8]

Published Information When diluted in glucose 5% or sodium chloride 0.9%, ciprofloxacin has been reported to be stable for 14 days at room temperature or in a refrigerator when protected from light.[5] No loss of ciprofloxacin 1.5mg/mL was observed by HPLC in 48 hours at 25°C in glucose 5% or sodium chloride 0.9% under fluorescent light.[9]

A solution comprising ciprofloxacin 2.86mg/mL in glucose 5% or sodium chloride 0.9% was found by HPLC to be stable for 90 days at 5°C or 25°C. The admixtures showed no change in appearance or pH throughout the study period.[10]

The stability of ciprofloxacin 0.025mg/mL (25mg/L) in peritoneal dialysis solutions containing glucose 1.5% and glucose 4.25% and stored for 14 days at 4°C, seven days at 25°C, or two days at 37°C was investigated by HPLC and UV spectrophotometry. Significant losses (4–10%) of ciprofloxacin were noted within the first 12 hours following the addition of the drug. Little further degradation was observed over the remaining study period. It was suggested that this initial loss was due to interaction with the plastic material of the container. The results supported a shelf-life of seven days for ciprofloxacin injection at 25°C in peritoneal dialysis solutions containing glucose 1.5% or glucose 4.25% with calcium 3.5mmol/2L and magnesium 1.5mmol/2L. In CAPD solutions based on glucose 4.25%, ciprofloxacin was stable for 48 hours at 37°C.[6]

In a similar study, losses of 0.76% at 4°C, 1.02% at 20°C, and 0.75% at 37°C were observed for a solution containing ciprofloxacin 50mg in 2L of a peritoneal dialysis solution with glucose 1.36%.[11]

Incompatibilities The solubility of ciprofloxacin decreases as the pH rises, therefore incompatibility is likely with high pH drug products such as aminophylline.[9]

Ciprofloxacin solutions have been reported to be physically or chemically incompatible with the following drug substances: aminophylline; amoxicillin; co-amoxiclav; cefepime hydrochloride; clindamycin phosphate; dexamethasone phosphate; flucloxacillin; frusemide; heparin sodium; hydrocortisone sodium succinate; magnesium sulphate; methylprednisolone; metronidazole; mezlocillin sodium; perfloxacin; sodium bicarbonate; and teicoplanin.[2,9,12-15]

Compatibilities Ciprofloxacin has been reported to be compatible with fructose 10%, glucose 5%, glucose 10%, glucose 4% with sodium chloride 0.18%, Ringer's solution, and sodium chloride 0.9%.[1]

Mixed combinations of ciprofloxacin 2mg/mL with gentamicin 12mg/mL or tobramycin 12mg/mL in glucose 5% or sodium chloride 0.9% were found by HPLC and immunoassay to be stable for at least 48 hours at 4°C or 25°C under fluorescent light. In the same study, a solution of ciprofloxacin 200mg/100mL mixed with metronidazole 500mg/100mL infusion and stored in a PVC bag, was found to be chemically stable for 48 hours at 25°C.[9]

A mixed solution of amikacin 4mg/mL and ciprofloxacin 1.5mg/mL in glucose 5% was stable for at least eight hours at 4°C, but less than 24 hours based on the amikacin assay. The same admixture at 25°C was stable for at least 48 hours.[9]

Physical compatibility of ciprofloxacin 1mg/mL or 2mg/mL (as lactate) with sodium bicarbonate solutions is variable. In sodium chloride 0.9% this combination is incompatible at all concentrations, but in glucose 5% some admixtures were reported to

be visually compatible during simulated Y-site administration.[13]

Comments

In common clinical practice, ciprofloxacin infusion in glucose 5% or sodium chloride 0.9% is stable for at least 14 days when stored at 4°C and at room temperature when protected from light. Information on physical compatibility should be interpreted with care.

References

1. ABPI. Compendium of data sheets and summaries of product characteristics 1996-1997. London: Datapharm Publications Ltd, 1996: 106-8.
2. Reynolds JEF, editor. Martindale: the extra pharmacopoeia, 31st edition. London: The Pharmaceutical Press, 1996: 207-10.
3. Ciproxin Flexibags. Pharm J 1997; 258: 711.
4. McEvoy GK, editor. American hospital formulary service drug information 1997. Bethesda, MD: American Society of Health-System Pharmacists Inc, 1997: 574-87.
5. Lomaestro BM, Bailie GR. Quinolone—cation interactions: a review. DICP Ann Pharmacother 1991; 11: 1249-58.
6. Kane MP, et al. Stability of ciprofloxacin injection in peritoneal dialysis solutions. Am J Hosp Pharm 1994; 51: 373-7.
7. Faouzi MA, et al. Stability and compatibility studies of pefloxacin, ofloxacin and ciprofloxacin with PVC infusion bags. Int J Hosp Pharm 1993; 89: 125-8.
8. Matsumoto M, et al. Photostability and biological activity of fluoroquinolones substituted at the 8-position after UV irradiation. Antimicrob Agents Chemother 1992; 36(8): 1715-9.
9. Goodwin SD, et al. Compatibility of ciprofloxacin injection with selected drugs and solutions. Am J Hosp Pharm 1991; 48: 2166-77.
10. Mathew M, Das Gupta V, Zerai T. The stability of ciprofloxacin in 5% dextrose and normal saline injections. J Clin Pharm Ther 1994; 19(4): 261-2.
11. Mahwhinney WM, et al. Stability of ciprofloxacin in peritoneal dialysis solution. Am J Hosp Pharm 1992; 49: 2956-9.
12. Trissel LA. Handbook on injectable drugs, 9th edition. Bethesda, MD: American Society of Health-System Pharmacists Inc, 1996: 271-4.
13. Gilbert DL, Trissel LA, Martinez JF. Compatibility of ciprofloxacin lactate with sodium bicarbonate during simulated Y-site administration. Am J Health-Syst Pharm 1997; 54: 1193-5.
14. Jim KL. The physical and chemical stability of intravenous ciprofloxacin with other drugs. Ann Pharmacother 1993; 27(6): 704-7.
15. Lyall D, Blythe J. Ciprofloxacin lactate infusion (letter). Pharm J 1987; 238: 290.

Prepared by

Tim Sizer

Clarithromycin

Approved Name
Clarithromycin

UK Proprietary Name
Klaricid (Abbott Laboratories Ltd)

Other Names
—

Product Details
Vials containing 500 mg of clarithromycin as a sterile, white, lyophilised powder. Vials also contain lactobionic acid as a solubilising agent.[1] The sodium content is negligible.

Preparation of Injection
When added to a 500 mg vial of clarithromycin, 10 mL of water for injection produces a solution containing 50 mg/mL of clarithromycin. This solution must be further diluted before intravenous administration.

For intravenous infusion, a solution containing clarithromycin 500 mg/250 mL should be prepared. Suitable infusion fluids are: compound sodium lactate; glucose 5%; glucose 5% in compound sodium lactate; glucose 5% in sodium chloride 0.3%; glucose 5% in sodium chloride 0.45%; and sodium chloride 0.9%.[1]

Administration
Clarithromycin 2 mg/mL should be administered by intravenous infusion over 60 minutes.[1] Clarithromycin should not be given as a bolus or intramuscular injection.

Stability in Practice
Clarithromycin vials should be stored at less than 30°C protected from light. In solution, clarithromy-cin degrades to decladinosyl-6-O-methyl-erythromycin A.

The manufacturer recommends that reconstituted solutions containing clarithromycin 50 mg/mL should be used within 24 hours of preparation. Solutions can be stored at temperatures of 5–25°C. Clarithromycin 2 mg/mL infusions should be used within six hours of preparation if stored at room temperature (25°C), or within 24 hours if stored at 5°C.[1]

Unpublished Information A clarithromycin 2 mg/mL infusion in sodium chloride 0.9% stored at 5°C is said to be stable for seven days.[2]

Incompatibilities Clarithromycin has been reported to be chemically or physically incompatible with the following drug substances: aminophylline; cefuroxime; flucloxacillin; frusemide; heparin; and phenytoin.[3]

Compatibilities Little information is available on the compatibility of clarithromycin with other drug substances. Information on physical compatibility should be interpreted with care.

Comments
Little information is available on the stability and compatibility of clarithromycin. The manufacturers recommendations should be followed.

References
1. ABPI. Compendium of data sheets and summaries of product characteristics 1996-1997. London: Datapharm Publications Ltd, 1996: 11.
2. Abbott Laboratories Ltd. Personal communication, 1996.
3. Taylor A. A physical compatibility study of clarithromycin injection with other commonly used injectable drugs. Pharm in Pract 1997; 7(9): 473-6.

Prepared by
Jeff Koundakjian

Clindamycin

Approved Name
Clindamycin

UK Proprietary Name
Dalacin C Phosphate (Pharmacia & Upjohn Ltd)

Other Names
—

Product Details
Clindamycin is available in glass ampoules containing 2 mL and 4 mL of a clear, colourless, sterile aqueous solution of clindamycin phosphate equivalent to 150 mg/mL of clindamycin base. Benzyl alcohol and disodium edetate are also included.[1]

The injection has a pH of 6.0–6.3 and an osmolality of 850 mosmol/kg.

Preparation of Injection
The injection is ready-to-use for intramuscular injection, but must be diluted for intravenous use (*see* below).

Administration
Clindamycin may be administered by either intramuscular or intravenous injection. Intravenous doses should be diluted with either glucose 5% or sodium chloride 0.9% and administered over 10–60 minutes.[1]

Stability in Practice
The commercial product has a shelf-life of 24 months when stored below 25°C; it should not be refrigerated.[1]

In aqueous solution, clindamycin is hydrolysed, the rate and mechanism of hydrolysis being dependent upon pH. Above pH 5, lincomycin, from which clindamycin is synthesised, is the major degradation product. However, between pH 0.4–4, the major degradation products are 1-dethiomethyl-1-hydroxy clindamycin and methyl mercaptan.[2] Clindamycin disappeared from reaction mixtures by an apparent first-order process under all of the conditions studied. In a study of clindamycin phosphate hydrolysis, clindamycin base is reported to be a lesser degradation product;[3] clindamycin phosphate itself was most stable in solution at pH 3.5–6.5.[4]

Published Information The commercial product was diluted to a final nominal concentration of 6 mg/mL, 9 mg/mL, and 12 mg/mL with glucose 5% and sodium chloride 0.9%, and studied under various storage conditions using reverse phase HPLC. Clindamycin phosphate was found to be stable for eight weeks at -10°C, 32 days at 4°C, and 16 days at 25°C, in glass and PVC containers, at all concentrations studied.[5]

In another study, clindamycin phosphate 300 mg was added to glucose 5% in PVC minibags, which were then frozen at -20°C for 30 days, then thawed and assayed for clindamycin content; the solutions retained over 90% of their potency for 24 hours after thawing.[6] This is in line with the results of a similar study in which clindamycin diluted to 6 mg/mL and 12 mg/mL in glucose 5% and sodium chloride 0.9% in PVC bags was shown to be stable for at least 22 days at 25°C, 54 days at 5°C, and 68 days at -10°C.[7]

The stability of clindamycin in polyolefin containers has also been studied. This showed that clindamycin 750 mg/mL in glucose 5% retained at least 90% of its potency after freezing for 30 days at -20°C, followed by 14 days in a refrigerator.[8]

Unpublished Information The stability of the commercial product has been investigated when stored in polypropylene syringes. Aliquots of the clindamycin phosphate were assayed by HPLC; 95% of the initial concentration of clindamycin 900 mg/6 mL was said to have been retained after 48 hours.[9] Various concentrations of clindamycin phosphate were said to be physically and chemically stable for 30 days when stored under fluorescent lighting at 25°C in disposable plastic syringes; the commercial product was diluted with water for injection to final concentrations of 20 mg/mL, 40 mg/mL, 60 mg/mL, and 120 mg/mL. The change in clindamycin concentration was small, ranging from 1.67–4.92%.[9]

Clindamycin phosphate 10 mg/mL in sodium chloride 0.9% was reported to be stable in an elastomeric device for 24 hours at room temperature or ten days if refrigerated.[10]

Incompatibilities   Solutions of clindamycin salts have a low pH, and incompatibilities can therefore be expected with alkaline preparations or drug substances unstable at low pH. Incompatibilities with the following drug substances have been reported: ampicillin sodium; aminophylline; barbiturates; calcium gluconate; ceftriaxone sodium; idarubicin hydrochloride; magnesium sulphate; phenytoin sodium; and ranitidine hydrochloride.[9]

Incompatibility with natural rubber has also been reported.

Compatibilities   Clindamycin is reported to be physically and chemically compatible for at least 24 hours in glucose 5% and sodium chloride 0.9% with the following drug substances at the usually administered concentrations: amikacin sulphate; aztreonam; cefotaxime sodium; cefoxitin sodium; ceftazidime sodium; ceftizoxime sodium; cephamandole nafate; cephazolin sodium; gentamicin sulphate; netilmicin sulphate; piperacillin; and tobramycin.[9,11,12]

Comments

In common clinical practice, clindamycin is stable when diluted in glucose 5% and sodium chloride 0.9%, and stored for 24 hours at room temperature.

None of the hydrolytic degradation products of clindamycin phosphate, under the storage conditions cited, have been reported to be toxic.

Studies have been published on the stability of clindamycin when mixed in the same intravenous infusion fluid with cephalosporins and with aminoglycosides; there are reports on the stability of admixtures of clindamycin with many, but not all, of these drugs, and information on any specific combination must be consulted.

The compatibility and duration of stability of drug admixtures will vary depending upon concentration and other conditions.

References

1. ABPI. Compendium of data sheets and summaries of product characteristics 1996-1997. London: Datapharm Publications Ltd, 1996: 764-765.
2. Oesterling TO. Aqueous stability of clindamycin. J Pharm Sci 1970; 59: 63-7.
3. Richards S, Lee MG, Parry P. Stability of clindamycin topical lotion. Proc Guild 1985; 20: 31-6.
4. Oesterling TO, Rowe EL. Hydrolysis of lincomycin-2-phosphate and clindamycin-2-phosphate. J Pharm Sci 1970; 59: 175-9.
5. Porter WR, et al. Compatibility and stability of clindamycin phosphate with intravenous fluids. Am J Hosp Pharm 1983; 40: 91-4.
6. Holmes JC, et al. Effect of freezing and microwave thawing on the stability of six antibiotic admixtures in plastic bags. Am J Hosp Pharm 1982; 39: 104-8.
7. Das Gupta V, et al. Stability of clindamycin phosphate in dextrose and saline solutions. Can J Hosp Pharm 1989; 42: 109-12.
8. Sarkar MA, et al. Stability of clindamycin phosphate, ranitidine hydrochloride and piperacillin sodium in polyolefin containers. Am J Hosp Pharm 1991; 48: 2184-6.
9. Pharmacia & Upjohn. Personal communication, 1997.
10. Block Medical Inc. Personal communication, 1996.
11. Foley PT, et al. Compatibility of clindamycin phosphate with cefotaxime sodium or netilmicin sulfate in small-volume admixtures. Am J Hosp Pharm 1985; 42: 839-43.
12. Mansur JM, et al. Stability and cost analysis of clindamycin-gentamicin admixtures given every eight hours. Am J Hosp Pharm 1985; 42: 332-5.

Prepared by

Ian Marsha

Co-amoxiclav

Approved Name
Co-amoxiclav

UK Proprietary Name
Augmentin Intravenous (SmithKline Beecham)

Other Names
Amoxycillin and clavulanic acid.

Product Details
Vials containing co-amoxiclav 600mg (amoxycillin 500mg/clavulanic acid 100mg) or co-amoxiclav 1.2g (amoxycillin 1g/clavulanic acid 200mg). The injection consists of a sterile powder of amoxycillin sodium and potassium clavulanate for reconstitution. Each 1.2g vial contains approximately 3.1mmol of sodium and 1.0mmol of potassium.[1] The reconstituted injection has a pH of 8.5–9.5.[2]

Preparation of Injection
The injection may be reconstituted by dissolving a 600mg vial in 10mL of water for injection, to produce a final volume of 10.5mL, or by dissolving a 1.2g vial in 20mL of water for injection, to produce a final volume of 20.9mL.

If more accurate reconstitution is required (e.g. for paediatric use) the following powder displacement value may be used: 0.5mL/600mg.[3]

Administration
Co-amoxiclav may be administered by intravenous injection over 3–4 minutes or by intravenous infusion over 30–40 minutes.

For infusion, a reconstituted 600mg vial should be further diluted in 50mL of fluid while the 1.2g vial should be diluted in 100mL of fluid. Suitable infusion fluids are: compound sodium lactate; potassium chloride and sodium chloride 0.9%; Ringer's solution; sodium chloride 0.9%; and water for injection.

Stability in Practice
The manufacturer recommends that the intravenous injection should be administered within 20 minutes of reconstitution, and that infusions are completed within four hours of reconstitution.[1] Infusions containing glucose, dextran or bicarbonate are less stable.

Satisfactory antibiotic concentrations are retained at 5°C and a reconstituted co-amoxiclav solution may be added to pre-refrigerated infusion bags and stored for up to eight hours. Thereafter, the infusion should be administered immediately after reaching room temperature.

Published Information The chemical stability of co-amoxiclav injection was investigated in a number of infusion fluids stored in PVC bags.[2] Analysis of amoxycillin was by HPLC and for clavulanic acid by HPLC and an imidazole chemical analysis. Various drug concentrations were used and storage was at 25°C, 5°C and -20°C (the latter being thawed by microwave radiation).

Stability was found to be highly concentration dependent with the clavulanate component being less stable than the amoxycillin. Stability increased with decreasing concentration. Co-amoxiclav 10mg/mL in sodium chloride 0.9% was reported to be stable for four hours at 25°C.[2]

Stability in sodium chloride 0.9% and water for injection was found to be enhanced by refrigeration. When stored at 4°C co-amoxiclav 10mg/mL was stable for 12.5 hours. Co-amoxiclav stability was also much lower in solutions containing glucose, dextran, or bicarbonate, with 90% of initial clavulanate activity being maintained for only 1–2 hours when using glucose 5% stored at 4°C before and after dilution. Aqueous solutions frozen at -20°C and thawed by microwave radiation lost more activity than those stored at 25°C.[2]

Unpublished Information Co-amoxiclav and heparin are said to be physically compatible if mixed together for a minimal period of time.[4]

Incompatibilities Studies of the compatibility of co-amoxiclav with quinolones have shown precipitation with both ciprofloxacin and perfloxacin.[5] A combination of gentamicin and co-amoxiclav was also observed to be chemically incompatible due to rapid decomposition of the gentamicin.[6]

Compatibilities The combination of metronidazole with co-amoxiclav has been found to be physically and chemically stable over a period of two hours, with the stability of clavulanic acid being the limiting factor.[7]

Comments

Co-amoxiclav stability is governed by the stability of clavulanic acid and is dependent on temperature, concentration, and diluent. The undiluted injection is only stable for about 20 minutes at room temperature, and diluents containing glucose will not maintain stability for more than 30 minutes. It is therefore important that close attention is paid to the reconstitution and administration of co-amoxiclav injection, and that administration guidelines are followed.

References

1. ABPI. Compendium of data sheets and summaries of product characteristics 1996-1997. London: Datapharm Publications Ltd, 1996: 115-6.

2. Ashwin J, Lynn B, Taskis CB. Stability and administration of intravenous Augmentin. Pharm J 1987; 238: 116-8.

3. Mulholland P. Displacement values of powder injections. Pharm J 1993; 251: 14-5.

4. SmithKline Beecham. Personal communication, 1995.

5. Janknegt R, et al. Quinolones and penicillins incompatibility. Drug Intell Clin Pharm 1989; 23: 91-2.

6. Janknegt R, et al. Which antibiotics can be combined in one infusion? Ziekenhuisfarmacie 1987; 3: 28-30.

7. Strehl E, Heni J. Physical and chemical compatibility and stability of a combination of amoxicillin/clavulanate potassium and metronidazole. Krankenhauspharmazie 1994; 15(10): 592-5.

Prepared by

Steve Brown

Co-trimoxazole

Approved Name
Co-trimoxazole

UK Proprietary Name
Septrin (Glaxo Wellcome)

Other Names
Trimethoprim and sulphamethoxazole.

Product Details
The proprietary preparation (Septrin infusion) contains co-trimoxazole equivalent to 80mg trimethoprim and 400mg sulphamethoxazole in each 5mL ampoule. The infusion is a faintly yellow coloured aqueous solution and contains 45% propylene glycol together with ethanol. It has a pH of approximately 10.[1] The osmolalities of co-trimoxazole in concentrations of 4.8mg/mL and 9.6mg/mL in glucose 5% were determined to be 541mosmol/kg and 798 mosmol/kg respectively. At a concentration of 9.6mg/mL in sodium chloride 0.9% the osmolality was determined to be 833mosmol/kg.[2]

Another preparation (Faulding Pharmaceuticals) contains 96mg/mL of co-trimoxazole in a 40% propylene glycol vehicle. The solution is clear and has a pH of approximately 10. It is available as either co-trimoxazole 480mg/5mL or 960mg/10mL in clear, glass ampoules.

Preparation of Injection
Co-trimoxazole must be diluted in an infusion solution before use. It should be added to an appropriate infusion fluid and shaken vigorously to ensure complete mixing. If visible turbidity or crystallisation appears at any time before or during infusion, the mixture should be discarded.[1]

Infusions may be prepared by adding either 5mL of co-trimoxazole to 125mL, 10mL to 250mL, or 20mL to 500mL of a compatible infusion fluid. Suitable infusion fluids are: dextran 40 10% in glucose 5% or sodium chloride 0.9%; dextran 70 6% in glucose 5% or sodium chloride 0.9%; glucose 5%; glucose 10%; Ringer's solution; sodium chloride 0.9%; and sodium chloride 0.18% and glucose 4%.[1]

Administration
Co-trimoxazole must be diluted prior to administration. It should be administered intravenously only in the form of an infusion solution, and may not be injected undiluted either intravenously or directly into an infusion line. Infusions should be administered over 1–1.5 hours, although this should be balanced against the fluid requirements of the patient.[1]

In situations where fluid restriction is necessary, co-trimoxazole may be administered at higher concentration than usual, and 5mL diluted with 75mL of glucose 5% has been used. Such a solution whilst being clear to the naked eye may on occasion exceed the BP limits set for particulate matter in large volume parenterals. The solution should be infused over a period not exceeding one hour. Any unused diluted solution should be discarded.[1]

The manufacturer recommends that no other agents are added to or mixed with a co-trimoxazole infusion.[1]

Stability In Practice
Undiluted co-trimoxazole solution should be stored at room temperature, protected from light; it should not be refrigerated. If stored at low temperatures, precipitation may occur, in which case the solution should be discarded.[2]

The solubility of trimethoprim in aqueous solutions is partially dependent on the pH of the solution. Trimethoprim is a weak base and its solubility is lower in solutions with a more alkaline pH.[2]

Diluted solutions should be used immediately as precipitation can occur at varying time periods.[2]

Published Information Co-trimoxazole solutions containing the equivalent of 3.84–4.8mg/mL in glucose 5% (1 in 20 dilution) are reported to be stable for four hours at room temperature. A 1 in 15 dilution in glucose 5% (4.8–6.4mg/mL) is reported to be stable for two hours at room temperature.[3]

A study of co-trimoxazole injection in five intravenous fluids suggested that dilutions of 1 in 25, 1 in 20, 1 in 15, and 1 in 10 were stable in all admixtures for 24 hours.[4] However, in a later study using similar dilutions it was reported that co-trimoxazole was stable in all concentrations studied in glucose 5% for 48 hours, but in sodium chloride 0.9% only a 1 in 25 dilution (3.84 mg/mL) was stable for 48 hours. More concentrated solutions were reported to be stable for much shorter periods and should be examined for signs of precipitation before use.[5]

Unpublished Information   Co-trimoxazole 960 mg/125 mL is said to be stable for 64 hours in glucose 5%, sodium chloride 0.9%, and glucose 4% with sodium chloride 0.18%, stored in PVC infusion bags at 25°C, protected from light.

Co-trimoxazole is also said to be stable for 48 hours in glucose 5% at a concentration of 1920 mg/125 mL in PVC infusion bags at 25°C, protected from light. At the same concentration, co-trimoxazole was said to be stable for 64 hours in sodium chloride 0.9%, under the same conditions.

Incompatibilities   There is little published information on the compatibility of co-trimoxazole with other drug substances. The manufacturers do not recommend admixing co-trimoxazole intravenous solutions with other drugs because of the potential for incompatibility.[1,3]

Compatibilities   Specialist references should be consulted for specific compatibility information.[2]

Comments

In common clinical practice, co-trimoxazole infusions should be prepared and administered within two hours because of the potential for precipitation. Solutions should not be refrigerated.

References

1. ABPI. Compendium of data sheets and summaries of product characteristics 1996-1997. London: Datapharm Publications Ltd, 1996: 1209-12.
2. Trissel LA. Handbook on injectable drugs, 9th edition. Bethesda, MD: American Society of Health-System Pharmacists Inc, 1996: 1063-8.
3. McEvoy GK, editor. American hospital formulary service drug information 1997. Bethesda, MD: American Society of Health-System Pharmacists Inc, 1997: 644-52.
4. Deans KW, Lang JR, Smith DE. Stability of trimethoprim-sulfamethoxazole injection in five infusion fluids. Am J Hosp Pharm 1982; 39: 1681-4.
5. Jarosinski PF, Kennedy PE, Gallelli JF. Stability of concentrated trimethoprim-sulfamethoxazole admixtures. Am J Hosp Pharm 1989; 46: 732-7.

Prepared by

Adele Jones

Diamorphine

Approved Name
Diamorphine hydrochloride

UK Proprietary Name
None (Suppliers: Berk, CP, Evans, and Hillcross.)

Other Names
Acetomorphine hydrochloride; diacetylmorphine hydrochloride; heroin hydrochloride.

Product Details
Clear, glass ampoules containing 5, 10, 30, 100 or 500 mg of diamorphine hydrochloride as a lyophilised powder. The powder has a negligible displacement value.[1]

When reconstituted with glucose 5% the injection has a pH of 3.8–4.4.

Preparation of Injection
Lyophilised diamorphine hydrochloride should be reconstituted with glucose 5%, sodium chloride 0.9%, or water for injection (minimum volume 1 mL for up to 100 mg and 2 mL for 500 mg). Reconstituted injections can be further diluted with glucose 5% or sodium chloride 0.9%, although glucose 5% is preferred.

Administration
Diamorphine hydrochloride may be administered by a variety of routes including intramuscular, intravenous, and subcutaneous injection. Continuous subcutaneous and intravenous infusion over 24–48 hours may also be used.[1,2]

Stability in Practice
Ampoules should be protected from light, stored below 25°C, and should not be used if the plug of powder is glassy or brown in colour or if the reconstituted solution is dark yellow. The commercially available products have a shelf-life of three years.

Diamorphine is incompatible with mineral acids, alkalis and chlorocresol.[3] The alkalinity of glass containers may be a contributory factor in the decomposition of solutions.

Diamorphine is relatively unstable in aqueous solution, and is hydrolysed to 3-*O*-monoacetylmorphine and 6-*O*-monoacetylmorphine and then to morphine;[4] however, 3-*O*-monoacetylmorphine is only occasionally detected. Hydrolysis takes place both in the dark and in the cold, and is associated with a fall in pH and development of an acetic odour.[5] The rate of degradation increases uniformly with temperature and initial concentration,[5] and is greatly increased at neutral or basic pH or with increased ionic strength.[6] Very small increases in ionic strength cause very large decreases in shelf-life and have a far greater effect than does pH on stability.[6]

Maximum shelf-life is achieved when no buffer is present; maximum stability occurs at pH 3.8–4.4.[3,7] Diamorphine hydrochloride exhibits a pH-dependent incompatibility in sodium chloride 0.9%. To remain in solution, the pH must be less than pH 6, particularly for diamorphine concentrations of 5 mg/mL or above.[8,9]

Diamorphine hydrochloride (0.3–200 mg/mL) is compatible with glucose 5% and sodium chloride 0.9% intravenous infusions, with aqueous solutions stable for 48 hours at pH 3.8–4.4, stability decreasing as the pH rises. For this reason, glucose 5% is the preferred diluent, as the pH of sodium chloride 0.9% may vary from 4.5–7.0.

Published Information   A variety of studies have been performed to determine the stability of diamorphine hydrochloride stored in syringes. In plastic syringes, the stability of a diamorphine 1 mg/mL solution was at least 28 days at 2–5°C and 26 days at room temperature.[10] At 2–20 mg/mL in water for injection, stability was 18 days at room temperature.[11]

In disposable glass syringes, diamorphine stability at 1 and 20 mg/mL concentration in sodium chloride 0.9% was 15 days at 4°C, and seven days at room temperature, respectively.[12]

Diamorphine hydrochloride 5 mg/mL in water for injection has been reported to be stable for 14 days at 4°C and 37°C in medication pump reservoirs.[13] Diamorphine infusions (1 and 20 mg/mL in sodium chloride 0.9%) in PVC bags and two disposable infusion devices were found to be stable for 15 days at

4°C and room temperature, and were also stable for 15 days at 31°C in both infusion devices, with the exception of the 1 mg/mL concentration in one infusion device which was only stable for 48 hours at 31°C.[12]

Solutions of diamorphine hydrochloride 250 mg/mL in sodium chloride 0.9% have been reported to be stable for 14 days during simulated patient use in a pump reservoir, and have been administered over seven days with no evidence of precipitation or irritation at the infusion site using syringe drivers and pump devices.[14]

Unpublished Information Diamorphine hydrochloride (0.2 and 2 mg/mL) in sodium chloride 0.9% or glucose 5% was said to be stable for 21 days at 4°C in PVC bags, although there was some loss due to adsorption (6 and 10%, respectively).[15] Diamorphine 5 mg/mL in water for injection in medication cassettes was said to be stable for 28 days at 4°C and seven days at 37°C.

The manufacturers recommend a shelf-life of 24 hours in plastic or glass syringes, or four hours in PVC bags, for solutions of diamorphine at concentrations of 10–50 mg/mL.

Incompatibilities Cyclizine (>10 mg/mL), is potentially incompatible with diamorphine (>10 mg/mL) in sodium chloride 0.9% at 25–37°C. Haloperidol (>1 mg/mL) is similarly potentially incompatible with diamorphine (>10 mg/mL) in sodium chloride 0.9% at 25–37°C, and these mixtures should not be used in slow infusion pumps.[16]

All solutions prepared in sodium chloride 0.9% should be checked daily for signs of precipitation, especially those intended for long-term infusions and those containing high concentrations of diamorphine, and it has been recommended that all diamorphine/antiemetic mixtures should be protected from light.[16]

Compatibilities Specialist references should be consulted for details of compatibility information, which should be interpreted with care.[17]

In PVC bags, bupivacaine hydrochloride 1.25 mg/mL is compatible with diamorphine hydrochloride 125 µg/mL in sodium chloride 0.9% for 28 days in the light at 25°C;[18] at 1.5 mg/mL bupivacaine hydrochloride is compatible with diamorphine 20 µg/mL in sodium chloride 0.9% for 20 days at 7°C, 12 days at 25–45°C, and six months at -18°C.[19] At 2.5 and 5 mg/mL in PVC bags, bupivacaine is compatible with diamorphine 0.5, 5, and

10 mg/mL for eight days at 25°C in the dark.[20]

Chlorpromazine 0.5 mg/mL is said to be compatible with diamorphine hydrochloride 0.3 and 1 mg/mL for four hours at 25°C in sodium chloride 0.9% in PVC bags. This mixture should not be administered by the subcutaneous route.

Cyclizine plus diamorphine mixtures are potentially incompatible, especially when the concentrations of either drug are >25 mg/mL. Solutions should be observed for any signs of precipitation before use, and it is not recommended that these mixtures are used in slow infusion pumps. However, the following mixtures have been shown to be compatible in plastic syringes: cyclizine 15 mg/mL plus diamorphine 15 mg/mL (24 hours at 25°C);[16] cyclizine 10 mg/mL plus diamorphine <20 mg/mL (24 hours at 5°C and 'in-use');[21] cyclizine 10 mg/mL plus diamorphine 10 mg/mL in water for injection (seven days at 25°C),[11] and cyclizine 6.7 mg/mL plus diamorphine 2–20 mg/mL or 100 mg/mL in water for injection (ten or seven days at 25°C, respectively).[11]

Dexamethasone 1.6 mg/mL is said to be compatible with diamorphine hydrochloride 10–50 mg/mL for 24 hours at 25–35°C.

Haloperidol plus diamorphine mixtures are potentially incompatible, particularly when the concentrations of haloperidol are >1 mg/mL. Solutions should be observed for any signs of precipitation before use, and it is not recommended that these mixtures are used in slow infusion pumps. At 0.75 mg/mL concentration, haloperidol is compatible with diamorphine hydrochloride 2, 20, and 100 mg/mL for 15 days, 21 days, and 24 hours, respectively, in plastic syringes at 25°C.[21]

Hyoscine butylbromide 20 mg/mL is compatible with diamorphine hydrochloride 50 and 150 mg/mL for seven days at 25°C in plastic syringes.[16]

Hyoscine hydrobromide 0.12 mg/mL is said to be compatible with diamorphine hydrochloride 10–50 mg/mL for 24 hours at 25–35°C in sodium chloride 0.9% in glass or plastic syringes, and at 0.4 mg/mL hyoscine hydrobromide is compatible with diamorphine hydrochloride 50 and 150 mg/mL for seven days in the dark at 25°C in plastic syringes.[16]

Methotrimeprazine 0.25 mg/mL is compatible with diamorphine hydrochloride 1 mg/mL in water for injection for 96 hours at 25°C in plastic syringes.[10] At 2.5 mg/mL concentration methotrimeprazine is said to be compatible with diamorphine hydrochloride 10mg/mL for 14 days at 30°C and 105 days at 4°C in sodium chloride 0.9% in plastic syringes, and at 10mg/mL it is said to be compatible with diamorphine hydrochloride 10–50mg/mL for 24 hours at 25–35°C, in sodium chloride 0.9% in glass or plastic syringes.

Metoclopramide 5mg/mL is said to be compatible with diamorphine hydrochloride 10–50mg/mL for 24 hours, and 50 or 150mg/mL for seven days,[16] in plastic syringes at room temperature, although a slight discoloration was observed after seven days.

Midazolam 0.67mg/mL is compatible with diamorphine hydrochloride 0.67mg/mL, and midazolam 5mg/mL is compatible with diamorphine hydrochloride 33.3mg/mL, for 14 days at 22°C in the dark in plastic syringes.[22]

Prochlorperazine 80µg/mL plus diamorphine hydrochloride 0.3 and 1mg/mL in sodium chloride 0.9% is said to be compatible for four hours at 25°C in glass and plastic syringes. This mixture should not be given by the subcutaneous route.

Comments

In common clinical practice, diamorphine infusion (1–200mg/mL) is stable for 48 hours in glucose 5% (the preferred diluent), sodium chloride 0.9%, and water for injection. In plastic syringes, the stability of 1–20mg/mL solutions is 18 days at 25°C, and in cassettes the stability of 5 and 20mg/mL infusions is 14 days under 'in-use' conditions.

Diamorphine is relatively unstable in aqueous solution, although the degradation products are thought to be the active species. The pH of maximum stability is 3.8–4.4; stability is greatly reduced with increased pH or increased ionic strength, and precipitation in sodium chloride 0.9% may occur above pH 5.6, especially at concentrations >5mg/mL.

Containers should be inspected for crystallisation prior to use, particularly when drug admixtures are to be administered. Information on physical compatibility must be interpreted with care.

References

1. ABPI. Compendium of data sheets and summaries of product characteristics 1996-1997. London: Datapharm Publications Ltd, 1996: 309-10.
2. Reynolds JEF, editor. Martindale: the extra pharmacopoeia, 31st edition. London: The Pharmaceutical Press, 1996: 34-6.
3. Davey EA, Murray JB. Hydrolysis of diamorphine in aqueous solutions. Pharm J 1969; 203: 737.
4. Lund W, editor. The pharmaceutical codex: principles and practice of pharmaceutics, 12th edition. London: The Pharmaceutical Press, 1994: 827-30.
5. Omar OA, et al. Diamorphine stability in aqueous solution for subcutaneous infusion. J Pharm Pharmacol 1989; 41: 275-27.
6. Beaumont IM. Stability study of aqueous solutions of diamorphine and morphine using HPLC. Pharm J 1982; 229: 39-41.
7. Allwood MC. Diamorphine mixed with antiemetic drugs in plastic syringes. Br J Pharm Pract 1984; 6: 88-90.
8. Kirk B, Hain WR. Diamorphine injection BP incompatibility. Pharm J 1985; 235: 171.
9. Page J, Hudson SA. Diamorphine hydrochloride compatibility with saline. Pharm J 1982; 228: 238-9.
10. Rogers GC, Davies MB, Allwood MC. An investigation into the stability of diamorphine hydrochloride with diazepam, metoclopramide or methotrimeprazine. Int Pharm J 1991; 5: 70.
11. Allwood MC. The stability of diamorphine alone and in combination with anti-emetics in plastic syringes. Palliative Med 1991; 5: 330-3.
12. Kleinberg ML, et al. Stability of heroin hydrochloride in infusion devices and containers for intravenous administration. Am J Hosp Pharm 1990; 47: 377-81.
13. Northcott M, et al. The stability of carboplatin, diamorphine, 5-fluorouracil and mitozantrone infusions in an ambulatory pump under storage and prolonged 'in-use' conditions. J Clin Pharm Ther 1991; 16: 123-9.
14. Jones VA, Hanks GW. New portable infusion pump for prolonged subcutaneous administration of opioid analgesics in patients with advanced cancer. Br Med J 1986; 292: 1496.
15. Adams P. Personal communication, 1996.
16. Regnard C, Pashley S, Westrope F. Anti-emetic/diamorphine mixture compatibility in infusion pumps. Br J Pharm Pract 1986; 8: 218-20.
17. Trissel LA. Handbook on injectable drugs, 9th edition. Bethesda, MD: American Society of Health-System Pharmacists Inc, 1996: 1129-31.
18. Grassby PF, Roberts DE. Stability of epidural opiate solutions in 0.9 per cent sodium chloride infusion bags. Int J Pharm Pract 1995; 3: 174-7.
19. Barnes AR, Nash S. Stability of bupivacaine hydrochloride with diamorphine hydrochloride in an epidural infusion. Pharm World Sci 1995; 17(3): 87-92.
20. Kreeger L, et al. Epidural diamorphine and bupivacaine stability study. Palliative Med 1995; 9: 315-8.
21. Allwood MC. The compatibility of high-dose diamorphine with cyclizine or haloperidol in plastic syringes. Int Pharm J 1991; 5: 120.
22. Allwood MC, Brown PW, Lee M. Stability of injections containing diamorphine and midazolam in plastic syringes. Int J Pharm Pract 1994; 3: 57-9.

Prepared by

Melanie Priston

Droperidol

Approved Name
Droperidol

UK Proprietary Name
Droleptan (Janssen-Cilag Ltd)

Other Names
—

Product Details
Commercially available as 2 mL glass ampoules containing droperidol 5 mg/mL. The injection also contains mannitol and lactic acid. The pH of the injection is pH 3.0–3.8 and the osmolality of a 2.5 mg/mL solution is 16 mosmol/kg.[1,2]

Preparation of Injection
Droperidol is in a ready-to-use form and may also be further diluted with the common intravenous infusion fluids.

Administration
Droperidol may be administered by intramuscular injection, slow intravenous injection, or intravenous infusion according to the manufacturers guidelines. The duration of action of droperidol is up to six hours.[1]

Stability in Practice
Droperidol appears to be stable under acidic conditions; it will precipitate at alkaline pH. Preparations should be protected from light.

Published Information   In a study of the stability of droperidol in compound sodium lactate, glucose 5%, and sodium chloride 0.9% infusions, droperidol was reported to be stable for seven days when stored in glass bottles. However, when a solution in compound sodium lactate was stored in PVC containers, there appeared to be some loss of droperidol due to sorption.[3]

Droperidol 0.2 mg/mL diluted in sodium chloride 0.9% was stored alone and in combination with morphine 2 mg/mL in 50 mL plastic syringes. Analysis by HPLC showed no loss of either drug, alone or in combination, after 14 days storage at room temperature in the light.[4]

Unpublished Information   An HPLC study of the stability of droperidol 0.05 mg/mL in polypropylene syringes with morphine sulphate 1 mg/mL in sodium chloride 0.9% found no significant degradation of either drug over six weeks at 4°C.[5]

Incompatibilities   Droperidol has been reported to be physically or chemically incompatible with the following drug substances: allopurinol;[6] fluorouracil; folinic acid; foscarnet;[7] frusemide; heparin; methohexitone; methotrexate; nafcillin sodium; piperacillin; thiopentone; and some barbiturates.[1,2]

Compatibilities   Specialist references should be consulted for specific compatibility information.[8]

Droperidol has been reported to be compatible in solution with morphine sulphate at a variety of concentrations.[4,5] Commercial products containing droperidol 2.5 mg/mL and fentanyl citrate 0.05 mg/mL are available in the US.[9]

Comments
In common clinical practice, droperidol is stable in sodium chloride 0.9% for at least seven days at room temperature.

References
1. ABPI. Compendium of data sheets and summaries of product characteristics 1996-1997. London: Datapharm Publications Ltd, 1996: 443-4.
2. Reynolds JEF, editor. Martindale: the extra pharmacopoeia, 31st edition. London: The Pharmaceutical Press, 1996: 707-8.
3. Ray JB, et al. Droperidol stability in intravenous admixtures. Am J Hosp Pharm 1983; 40: 94-7.
4. Williams OA, et al. Stability of morphine and droperidol, separately and combined, for use as an infusion. Hosp Pharm Pract 1992; 2(9): 597-600.
5. Neel A. Personal communication, 1995.
6. Trissel LA, Martinez JF. Physical compatibility of allopurinol sodium with selected drugs during simulated Y-site administration. Am J Hosp Pharm 1994; 51: 792-9.
7. Lor E, Takagi J. Visual compatibility of foscarnet with other injectable drugs. Am J Hosp Pharm 1990; 47: 157-9.
8. Trissel LA. Handbook on injectable drugs, 9th edition. Bethesda, MD: American Society of Health-System Pharmacists Inc, 1996: 390-5.
9. McEvoy GK, editor. American hospital formulary service drug information 1997. Bethesda, MD: American Society of Health-System Pharmacists Inc, 1997: 1833-5.

Prepared by
John Hubbard

Erythromycin

Approved Name
Erythromycin lactobionate

UK Proprietary Name
None (Suppliers: Abbott Laboratories Ltd; Faulding Pharmaceuticals.)

Other Names
—

Product Details
Commercially available in vials containing 1 g of erythromycin lactobionate as a sterile white lyophilised powder.[1,2] Sodium content is negligible.

Preparation of Injection
When added to a vial, 20 mL of water for injection provides 22 mL of solution; 20 mL of this solution contains 1 g of erythromycin lactobionate. The solution must be further diluted prior to intravenous administration.

The formation of a precipitate will result if sodium chloride 0.9% or other solutions containing inorganic ions are used in the preliminary reconstitution. The powder is slow to dissolve, requiring patience and vigorous agitation of the vial.

Infusions should be prepared by adding the reconstituted injection to sodium chloride 0.9% or neutralised glucose 5% solution according to the manufacturers guidelines.[1,2] Neutralised glucose 5% solution is prepared by adding 5 mL of sodium bicarbonate 8.4% to 1 L of glucose 5%.

Administration
Erythromycin may be administered by continuous intravenous infusion; the usual concentration of erythromycin lactobionate being 1 mg/mL (0.1%).[1,2]

Intermittent intravenous infusion in strengths up to 5 mg/mL may be given in volumes over 100 mL over 20–60 minutes and repeated at intervals not greater than every six hours.

Bolus and intramuscular injection is not recommended.

Stability in Practice
The degradation of erythromycin in aqueous solutions follows first-order kinetics and is dependent on pH. Erythromycin is particularly unstable at less than pH 5.5 or greater than pH 10.0. The stability of erythromycin solutions can be significantly improved if the pH of acidic intravenous fluids are raised by the addition of a buffer. Studies have also found that the rate of degradation increases as pH rises, due in part to a base catalysis reaction.[3-7]

Published Information Aqueous solutions of erythromycin lactobionate 50 mg/mL have a pH of 7 and are stable for two weeks when refrigerated at 2–8°C or for 24 hours at room temperature. Following further dilution of this concentrated solution to an erythromycin 1–5 mg/mL in sodium chloride 0.9% solution, stability is variable and depends on several factors including type of container, resultant pH, and temperature.[3-7] Because of the variability of specific stability information, the manufacturers recommend that, to ensure potency, all solutions for administration should be used within eight hours of preparation.[1,2]

Solutions containing erythromycin lactobionate 50 mg/mL in water for injection and further diluted with sodium chloride 0.9% to a 5 mg/mL or 4 mg/mL solution, and the pH adjusted to pH 7.5–8.0 using sodium bicarbonate 8.4% solution, were studied using an HPLC technique. Erythromycin lactobionate could be assigned a shelf-life of up to 60 days storage at 5°C. Unbuffered solutions should not be assigned a shelf-life of greater than 20 days to ensure all batches and concentrations retain greater than 95% of the added erythromycin.[3]

Analysis by a stability indicating HPLC method showed that injections prepared according to the manufacturers instructions, when stored at 5°C are relatively stable and can be assigned a shelf-life of two months.[4]

The stability of erythromycin lactobionate solution was not affected by storage for 12 months at -20°C followed by microwave thawing.[8]

Unpublished Information Erythromycin lactobionate reconstituted with water for injection to a concentration of 50mg/mL is said to be stable for 24 hours at room temperature in light and 14 days at 8°C.

Erythromycin lactobionate 1mg/mL is also said to be stable for 24 hours in sodium chloride 0.9%, buffered and unbuffered, and in neutralised glucose 5% solution.

Incompatibilities Erythromycin solutions have been reported to be physically or chemically incompatible with the following drug substances: amikacin; aminophylline; barbiturates; some cephalosporins such as cephalothin and cephazolin; chloramphenicol; colistin sulphomethate sodium; flucloxacillin; heparin sodium; metaraminol; metoclopramide; phenytoin; streptomycin; tetracyclines; and some vitamins.[9]

Compatibilities Specialist references should be consulted for specific compatibility information.[10] Information on physical compatibility should be interpreted with care.

Comments

Because of the variability of stability information, unbuffered solutions of erythromycin lactobionate should be used within eight hours of preparation.

References

1. ABPI. Compendium of data sheets and summaries of product characteristics 1996-1997. London: Datapharm Publications Ltd, 1996: 4.
2. ABPI. Compendium of data sheets and summaries of product characteristics 1996-1997. London: Datapharm Publications Ltd, 1996: 334-5.
3. Pluta PL, Morgan PK. Stability of erythromycin in intravenous admixtures. Am J Hosp Pharm 1986; 43: 2732, 2738.
4. Paesen J, et al. Study of the stability of erythromycin in neutral and alkaline solutions by liquid chromatography on poly(styrene-divinylbenzene). Int J Pharmaceutics 1994; 113: 215-22.
5. Allwood MC. The stability of erythromycin injection in small-volume infusions. Int J Pharmaceutics 1990; 62: R1-R3.
6. Allwood MC. The influence of buffering on the stability of erythromycin injection in small-volume infusions. Int J Pharmaceutics 1992; 80: R7-R9.
7. McEvoy GK, editor. American hospital formulary service drug information 1997. Bethesda, MD: American Society of Health-System Pharmacists Inc, 1997: 235-6.
8. Sewell GJ, Palmer AJ. The chemical and physical stability of three intravenous infusions subjected to frozen storage and microwave thawing. Int J Pharmaceutics 1991; 72: 57-63.
9. Reynolds JEF, editor. Martindale: the extra pharmacopoeia, 31st edition. London: The Pharmaceutical Press, 1996: 225-9.
10. Trissel LA. Handbook on injectable drugs, 9th edition. Bethesda, MD: American Society of Health-System Pharmacists Inc, 1996: 413-8.

Prepared by

Jeff Koundakjian

Fentanyl

Approved Name
Fentanyl

UK Proprietary Name
Sublimaze (Janssen-Cilag Ltd)

Other Names
—

Product Details
Fentanyl is available as a clear, colourless, aqueous injection presented in 2 mL and 10 mL ampoules. The injection contains fentanyl 50 µg/mL, as the citrate, in water for injection and sodium chloride.[1] The pH of the injection is 4–7.5.[2] Osmolality is determined to be essentially zero.

Preparation of Injection
See below.

Administration
Fentanyl may be administered by intramuscular or intravenous injection. Intravenously, it may be administered to both adults and children according to set dosage regimens. As a bolus injection, 10 mL of fentanyl gives analgesia lasting for about one hour.

Fentanyl may also be administered as an intravenous infusion in glucose 5% or sodium chloride 0.9%.

Stability in Practice
The manufacturer recommends that fentanyl infusions should be used within 24 hours of preparation.[1]

Published Information Fentanyl citrate 5 µg/mL in glucose 5% and sodium chloride 0.9% was found to be stable for 48 hours when stored in PVC infusion bags and glass containers at room temperature (22°C) in normal room light; the concentration of fentanyl delivered by a patient-controlled system was also relatively constant over a 30 hour study period.[3]

Fentanyl citrate 20 µg/mL in sodium chloride 0.9% has been reported to be stable for 30 days when stored at 3°C or 23°C in PVC reservoirs for portable infusion devices.[4]

Incompatibilities Fentanyl has been reported to be physically or chemically incompatible with the following drug substances: methohexitone; and thiopentone.[1]

Compatibilities Fentanyl is said to be compatible with most agents commonly used in anaesthesia.

An admixture of fentanyl citrate 20 µg/mL and bupivacaine hydrochloride 1.25 µg/mL in sodium chloride 0.9% in PVC containers (reservoirs for portable infusion devices) was found to be physically compatible and stable when stored for 30 days at 3°C or 23°C, with little or no loss of either drug.[5]

Fentanyl citrate 2 µg/mL with bupivacaine 1 mg/mL in sodium chloride 0.9% in PVC bags and polypropylene syringes was found to be stable for 12 weeks at room temperature in the light, and at 8°C.[6]

The physical and chemical stability of fentanyl 10 µg/mL in combination with bupivacaine 1.5 mg/mL and ketamine 2 mg/mL in sodium chloride 0.9% in polypropylene syringes was investigated by GC/MS. After one hour at room temperature no visible or chemical changes were detected. Similar results were reported for combinations of fentanyl 10 µg/mL, clonidine 30 µg/mL, and lignocaine 2 mg/mL in sodium chloride 0.9%.[7]

In another study,[8] the stability of solutions containing fentanyl, bupivacaine, and adrenaline, alone and in combination was studied over a period of 56 days when stored at various temperatures in the light or in the dark in PVC bags. Over the first three days of the study, both fentanyl and bupivacaine were adsorbed from solution onto the PVC, subsequently however, concentrations of both drugs remained relatively constant. There was no sign of precipitation in any of the solutions studied.

Comments
Studies indicate that fentanyl citrate 5 µg/mL in glucose 5% or sodium chloride 0.9% is stable when stored in glass or PVC containers at room temperature under normal light conditions for up to 48 hours, and that fentanyl citrate 20 µg/mL in sodium chloride 0.9% is stable and compatible when stored

in PVC portable infusion pump reservoirs for 30 days at 3°C and 23°C. However, data from these studies cannot be extrapolated to different solutions or different fentanyl concentrations because both stability and compatibility depends upon solution pH.

References

1. ABPI. Compendium of data sheets and summaries of product characteristics 1996-1997. London: Datapharm Publications Ltd, 1996: 472-3.
2. Reynolds JEF, editor. Martindale: the extra pharmacopoeia, 31st edition. London: The Pharmaceutical Press, 1996: 43-6.
3. Kowalski SR, Gourlay GK. Stability of fentanyl citrate in glass and plastic containers and in a patient-controlled delivery system. Am J Hosp Pharm 1990; 47: 1584-7.
4. Allen LV, Stiles ML, Tu Y-H. Stability of fentanyl citrate in 0.9% sodium chloride solution in portable infusion pumps. Am J Hosp Pharm 1990; 47: 1572-4.
5. Tu Y-H, Stiles MH, Allen LV. Stability of fentanyl citrate and bupivacaine hydrochloride in portable pump reservoirs. Am J Hosp Pharm 1990; 47: 2037-40.
6. Mehta AC, Petty DR. How stable are bupivacaine and fentanyl? Pharm in Pract 1995; 5(1): 21-2.
7. Christie JM, Jones CW, Markowsky SJ. Chemical compatibility of regional anaesthetic drug combinations. Ann Pharmacother 1992; 26: 1078-80.
8. Dawson PJ, et al. Stability of fentanyl, bupivacaine and adrenaline solutions for extradural infusion. Br J Anaesth 1992; 68: 414-7.

Prepared by

Mike Booth

Flucloxacillin

Approved Name
Flucloxacillin

UK Proprietary Name
Floxapen (SmithKline Beecham)

Other Names
Floxacillin.

Product Details
Vials of a dry powder for reconstitution containing 250 mg, 500 mg, and 1 g of flucloxacillin as the sodium salt. Also available as frozen infusion bags containing 500 mg, 1 g, and 2 g of flucloxacillin in sodium chloride 0.9%.

The pH of a 10% solution in water is 5–7. The sodium content is 1.13 mmol/500 mg vial.

Preparation of Injection
The powder has a displacement value of 0.4 mL/500 mg. Vials may be reconstituted with glucose 5%, sodium chloride 0.9%, or water for injection. The maximum volume of diluent that can be added to each vial is 9.8 mL for the 250 mg vial; 9.6 mL for the 500 mg vial; and 19.2 mL for the 1 g vial.

Administration
Flucloxacillin may be administered by intravenous injection over 3–5 minutes. Vials containing either 250 mg or 500 mg should be reconstituted with 5–10 mL of water for injection while the 1 g vial should be reconstituted with 15–20 mL of water for injection. Solutions containing 0.5–2 g may be similarly prepared and further diluted in a suitable diluent for administration over 5–20 minutes.[1,2]

It has been suggested that intermittent bolus infusion producing high antibiotic concentrations for comparatively short periods, has advantages over intravenous bolus injection.[1,2]

Stability in Practice
The susceptibility of penicillins to degradation in aqueous solutions is due to the lability of the beta-lactam ring. The rate of degradation increases with increasing temperature and inactivation is also promoted by conditions of high or low pH. In general, penicillins have a good degree of stability within the range pH 5.5–7.5. However, the initial slow decomposition leads to a fall in pH, which increases the rate of degradation.[3]

The commercially available frozen infusion bags are said to be stable for 90 days at -20°C; seven days at 4°C; and 24 hours at room temperature.

Solutions in glucose 5%, sodium chloride 0.9%, and water for injection are said to retain their activity for up to 72 hours.[4]

Published Information An unbuffered flucloxacillin 2% solution stored at 37°C for seven days was found to contain 35% of the degradation product *N*-formylpenicillamine.[5]

The results of a study using HPLC to investigate the stability of flucloxacillin sodium 0.5–2 g as an infusion in 100 mL of sodium chloride 0.9% suggested that by applying an arbitrary criteria of retention of 90% or more of the initial concentration, a shelf-life of 28 days, when stored in a refrigerator, could be allocated. However, it was suggested that due to the variability of pH and drug concentration in the infusion, a shelf-life of 21 days was more appropriate to allow more confidence in the suitability for use of the infusion at the end of the storage period.[6]

Another study investigating the stability of flucloxacillin in syringes suggested a seven day expiry at 4–8°C; analysis was by biological assay.[7]

Unpublished Information Two studies examining the stability of flucloxacillin 50 mg/mL stored in syringes suggested a shelf-life of three and seven days respectively when stored at 4°C.[8,9]

Incompatibilities Flucloxacillin should not be mixed with blood, proteins, or lipid emulsions, and should be administered separately from aminoglycosides.[10]

Flucloxacillin has been reported to be chemically or physically incompatible with the following drug substances: amiodarone; buprenorphine; calcium gluconate; chlorpromazine hydrochloride; ciprofloxacin; clarithromycin;[11] diazepam; dobutamine hydrochloride; erythromycin lactobionate; gentamicin sulphate; metoclopramide hydrochloride; morphine sulphate; netilmicin sulphate; ofloxacin;

papaveretum; pefloxacin; pethidine hydrochloride; prochlorperazine edisylate; promethazine hydrochloride; tobramycin; and verapamil hydrochloride.

Compatibilities   A study examining the compatibility of flucloxacillin with several commonly used drugs showed a high incidence of visual incompatibility.[12]

Comments

From the available data, flucloxacillin in sodium chloride 0.9% may be stable for seven days in a refrigerator or three days at room temperature.

References

1. Bergan T, Oydvin B. Crossover study of penicillin pharmacokinetics after intravenous infusions. Chemotherapy 1974; 20(5): 263-79.
2. Curcio L. Optimal dosage regimen for penicillins: bolus or continuous infusion? J Antimicrob Chemother 1979; 5: 503-9.
3. Lynn B. The stability and administration of intravenous penicillins. Br J Intraven Ther 1981; 2(3): 22-39.
4. SmithKline Beecham. Personal communication, 1996.
5. Bird AE, Jennings KR, Marshall AC. N-Formylpenicillamine and penicillamine as degradation products of penicillins in solution. J Pharm Pharmacol 1986; 38: 913-7.
6. McLaughlin JP, Simpson C, Taylor RA. When is flucloxacillin stable? Hosp Pharm Pract 1993; 3: 553-6.
7. Ahmed ST, Parkinson R. The stability of drugs in pre-filled syringes: flucloxacillin, ampicillin, cefuroxime, cefotaxime and ceftazidime. Hosp Pharm Pract 1992; 2: 285-9.
8. Shaw R. Personal communication, 1996.
9. Adams P, Haines-Nutt F. Personal communication, 1996.
10. ABPI. Compendium of data sheets and summaries of product characteristics 1996-1997. London: Datapharm Publications Ltd, 1996: 116-7.
11. Taylor A. A physical compatibility study of clarithromycin injection with other commonly used injectable drugs. Pharm in Pract 1997; 7(9): 473-6.
12. Beatson C, Taylor A. A physical compatibility study of frusemide and flucloxacillin injections. Br J Pharm Pract 1987; 9: 223-6, 236.

Prepared by

Chris Pritchard

Fluconazole

Approved Name

Fluconazole

UK Proprietary Name

Diflucan (Pfizer Ltd)

Other Names

—

Product Details

Commercially available as an intravenous infusion containing fluconazole 2 mg/mL in sodium chloride 0.9%. Available in 25 mL (50 mg) and 100 mL (200 mg) bottles.[1] The infusion has a pH of 5–7 and is iso-osmotic, with an osmolality of 300–315 mosmol/L.[2] Each 100 mL (200 mg) of fluconazole infusion contains 15 mmol of sodium.

Preparation of Injection

Bottles contain a solution ready-to-use for intravenous infusion.

Administration

Fluconazole may be administered by intravenous infusion at a rate of 5–10 mL/min. Where necessary, fluconazole can be further diluted in the following solutions: compound sodium lactate; glucose 20%; potassium chloride in glucose; Ringer's solution; sodium bicarbonate 4.2%; and sodium chloride 0.9%.[1]

Stability in Practice

Fluconazole is generally considered to be a stable substance, only degrading in concentrated sulphuric acid under reflux conditions.

The commercial fluconazole infusion should be stored at room temperature (below 30°C) and should not be frozen.[1]

Published Information Fluconazole 1 mg/mL infusion stored at 25°C under standard fluorescent light has been reported to be stable for 72 hours in potassium chloride plus glucose 5% injection, and in theophylline plus glucose 5% injection. In compound sodium lactate, fluconazole 1 mg/mL was sta-

ble for 24 hours under the same storage conditions.[3]

Unpublished Information Fluconazole 2 mg/mL was reported to be stable in an elastomeric infusion device for 24 hours at room temperature or 14 days in a refrigerator.[4]

Incompatibilities A simulated Y-site administration study suggested that fluconazole was visually incompatible with the following drug substances: amphotericin; cefotaxime; ceftazidime; ceftriaxone; cefuroxime; chloramphenicol; clindamycin; co-trimoxazole; diazepam; erythromycin; frusemide; haloperidol; hydroxyzine; imipenem with cilastatin; pentamidine; piperacillin; and ticarcillin.[5] Aciclovir and vancomycin showed no obvious signs of incompatibility.[5]

Compatibilities A simulated Y-site administration study showed that fluconazole 2 mg/mL was compatible with paclitaxel 0.3 mg/mL and 1.2 mg/mL for at least four hours when mixed in glass testtubes.[6]

A simulated Y-site study evaluating the chemical stability of fluconazole, ondansetron, and ranitidine showed that ranitidine 0.5 mg/mL or 2 mg/mL may be administered along with either fluconazole 2 mg/mL or ondansetron 0.03–0.3 mg/mL for up to four hours.[7]

Fluconazole 1 mg/mL has been reported to be chemically stable for 72 hours at 25°C under normal lighting conditions when mixed with the following drug substances: aciclovir sodium 10 mg/mL; amikacin sulphate 5 mg/mL; amphotericin B 0.1 mg/mL; cephazolin sodium 20 mg/mL; clindamycin phosphate 12 mg/mL; gentamicin sulphate 1 mg/mL; metronidazole hydrochloride 5 mg/mL; and piperacillin sodium 80 mg/mL.[8]

Comments

Fluconazole solutions should not be mixed with other drug substances. However, dilutions with glucose 5% or sodium chloride 0.9% may be stable for three days at room temperature.

References

1. ABPI. Compendium of data sheets and summaries of product characteristics 1996-1997. London: Datapharm Publications

Ltd, 1996: 744-6.

2. McEvoy GE, editor. American hospital formulary service drug information 1997. Bethesda, MD: American Society of Health-System Pharmacists Inc, 1997: 79-88.

3. Hunt-Fugate AK, Hennessey CK, Kazarian CM. Stability of fluconazole in injectable solutions. Am J Hosp Pharm 1990; 50: 1186-7.

4. Fresenius Healthcare Group. Personal communication, 1996.

5. Lor A, Sheybani T, Takagi J. Visual compatibility of fluconazole with commonly used injectable drugs during simulated Y-site administration. Am J Hosp Pharm 1991; 48: 744-6.

6. Burm J-P, et al. Stability of paclitaxel and fluconazole during simulated Y-site administration. Am J Hosp Pharm 1994; 51: 2704-6.

7. Pompilio FM, et al. Stability of ranitidine hydrochloride with ondansetron hydrochloride or fluconazole during simulated Y-site administration. Am J Hosp Pharm 1994; 51: 391-4.

8. Inagaki K, et al. Stability of fluconazole in commonly used intravenous antibiotic solutions. Am J Hosp Pharm 1990; 50: 1206-8.

Prepared by

Chris Pritchard

Foscarnet Sodium

Approved Name

Foscarnet sodium

UK Proprietary Name

Foscavir (Astra Pharmaceuticals Ltd)

Other Names

—

Product Details

Clear glass bottles (250 mL and 500 mL) containing foscarnet trisodium hexahydrate 24 mg/mL in water for injection. The solution is isotonic and adjusted to pH 7.4 with hydrochloric acid.[1] Sodium content is approximately 0.37 mmol/mL.

Preparation of Injection

The injection is presented in a ready-to-use form.

Administration

Foscarnet sodium injection should only be administered intravenously.

When infused via a peripheral vein, foscarnet sodium must be diluted with glucose 5% or sodium chloride 0.9% to a concentration of 12 mg/mL. However, foscarnet sodium may be administered undiluted via the central vein.

Stability in Practice

The injection should be stored below 30°C and not refrigerated. If refrigerated or exposed to temperatures below freezing point precipitation may occur. The precipitate can be brought back into solution by storing at room temperature with repeated shaking.

Foscarnet sodium injection and dilutions in equal parts with glucose 5% or sodium chloride 0.9% in PVC bags is stable for seven days.[1]

Published Information The stability of diluted foscarnet sodium solution has been investigated by stability indicating techniques. It has been reported that solutions containing foscarnet sodium 12 mg/mL in glucose 5% or sodium chloride 0.9% when stored in PVC bags are stable for 35 days at 5°C and 25°C (analysis by UV spectroscopy).[2]

Solutions containing foscarnet sodium 12 mg/mL in sodium chloride 0.9% when stored in PVC bags were stable when analysed by HPLC for 30 days at 25°C in light or dark and at 5°C in the dark.[3] Solutions remained clear and without significant changes in pH.

Solutions of foscarnet sodium 12 mg/mL in sodium chloride 0.9% were packaged in glass infusion bottles with rubber bungs and autoclaved at 121°C for 15 minutes. The solutions were assayed by HPLC and found to be stable to autoclaving.[4]

Unpublished Information Injections of foscarnet sodium 12 mg/mL diluted in sodium chloride 0.9% or 24 mg/mL (undiluted) are reported to be stable in an elastomeric infusion device for seven days at room temperature and 14 days in a refrigerator.[5]

Incompatibilities Foscarnet sodium injection is reported to be incompatible with the following drug substances: aciclovir sodium; amphotericin B; co-trimoxazole; diazepam; digoxin; diphenhydramine; dobutamine; droperidol; ganciclovir; glucose 30%; haloperidol; leucovorin; lorazepam; midazolam; pentamidine isethionate; phenytoin; prochlorperazine; promethazine; trimetrexate; and vancomycin.[1,6,7]

Additionally, foscarnet sodium may chelate divalent metal ions and is chemically incompatible with solutions containing calcium.

Compatibilities Foscarnet sodium is chemically and physically compatible with glucose 5% and sodium chloride 0.9% intravenous solutions.

Studies using a simulated Y-injection site in a 1:1 ratio have found the following drugs to be physically compatible with foscarnet sodium. Tests were carried out over a 24 hour period at room temperature under normal fluorescent room lighting. No chemical studies were carried out: amikacin sulphate; aminophylline; ampicillin sodium; aztreonam; benzquinamide hydrochloride; benzylpenicillin potassium; cefoperazone; cefoxitin sodium; ceftazidime; ceftizoxime sodium; cefuroxime; cephazolin sodium; chloramphenicol sodium succinate; cimetidine; clindamycin phosphate; dexamethasone sodium phosphate; dopamine hydrochloride; erythromycin lactobionate; fluconazole; frusemide; gentamicin sulphate; heparin sodium; hydrocortisone sodium succinate; hydromorphone hydrochloride; hydroxyzine hydrochloride; imipenem-cilastatin sodium; metoclopramide; metronidazole; miconazole; morphine sulphate; oxacillin sodium; phenytoin sodium; piperacillin sodium; and tobramycin sulphate.[6-8]

Comments

Foscarnet sodium 12 mg/mL infusions are stable in glucose 5% or sodium chloride 0.9% for at least 28 days at room temperature.

References

1. ABPI. Compendium of data sheets and summaries of product characteristics 1996-1997. London: Datapharm Publications Ltd, 1996: 73-4.
2. Mathew M, Das Gupta V, Bethea C. Stability of foscarnet sodium in 5% dextrose and 0.9% sodium chloride injections. J Clin Pharm Ther 1994; 19: 35-6.
3. Woods K, et al. Stability of foscarnet sodium in 0.9% sodium chloride injection. Am J Hosp Pharm 1994; 51: 88-90.
4. Trissel LA. Handbook on injectable drugs, 9th edition. Bethesda, MD: American Society of Health-System Pharmacists Inc, 1996: 483-7.
5. Fresenius Healthcare Group. Personal communication, 1996.
6. Baltz JK, et al. Visual compatibility of foscarnet with other injectable drugs during simulated Y-site administration. Am J Hosp Pharm 1990; 47: 2075-7.
7. Lor E, Takagi J. Visual compatibility of foscarnet with other injectable drugs. Am J Hosp Pharm 1990; 47: 157-9.
8. Lor E, Sheybani T, Takagi J. Visual compatibility of fluconazole with commonly used injectable drugs during simulated Y-site administration. Am J Hosp Pharm 1991; 48: 744-6.

Prepared by

Con Hanson

Frusemide

Approved Name

Frusemide

UK Proprietary Name

Lasix (Hoechst Marion Roussel Ltd)
A number of non-proprietary preparations are also available.

Other Names

Furosemide.

Product Details

Available as an injection, in amber glass ampoules, containing frusemide 20 mg/2 mL and 50 mg/5 mL with sodium chloride and sodium hydroxide. Frusemide 250 mg/25 mL contains mannitol and sodium hydroxide (sodium content is approximately 0.014 mmol/mL for the low strengths and 0.04 mmol/mL for the higher strengths).[1]

Frusemide Injection BP is also available at concentrations of 10 mg/mL, 20 mg/2 mL, and 50 mg/5 mL.

The pH of the BP injection is 8.0–9.3 and the osmolality is 287 mosmol/kg.

Preparation of Injection

See below.

Administration

Frusemide may be administered by intramuscular or slow intravenous injection at a rate not more than 4 mg/min.

Frusemide may also be administered by continuous intravenous infusion at a rate not more than 4 mg/min in sodium chloride 0.9% or Ringer's solution. Frusemide is less soluble at low pH. Solutions should be above pH 5.5, therefore glucose infusions are not usually suitable.[1] Rapid infusion may produce transient deafness.[2]

Stability in Practice

Frusemide injection 10 mg/mL has been reported to be stable for two months when stored in polypropylene syringes at 4°C and 25°C and protected from light. Less than 1% of saluamine (a principal degra-

dation product) was detected by HPLC analysis after two months.[3]

Frusemide injection 2 mg/mL has been found to be stable in glucose 5% and glucose 10% for 24 hours.[4]

Exposure to light may cause discoloration and solutions should not be used if a yellow colour has developed. Refrigeration may cause precipitation although resolubilisation may be carried out by warming at room temperature without affecting stability.[5]

Published Information Frusemide is significantly more soluble in alkaline solutions than in acid (*see* table), and is liable to precipitate in conditions of low pH.[6]

Solubility of frusemide (mg/100 mL)	pH
18	2.3
26	4.0
81	6.0
123	8.0
1336	10.0

The stability of frusemide in solution is pH dependent. In aqueous solution, frusemide undergoes an acid-catalysed hydrolysis to form saluamine and a furfuryl alcohol,[7] above pH 4 this reaction is slower and above pH 8 becomes negligible.[8]

At a concentration of 1 mg/mL in sodium chloride 0.9% infusion bags, frusemide has been shown to undergo no degradation after 24 hours at 25°C when exposed to light or in the dark. At 6°C, a 9.7% loss of frusemide was reported after 26 days.[9] A further study at frusemide concentrations of 200 µg/mL and 400 µg/mL showed a 5–7% loss in 24 hours at 25°C.[10]

Frusemide degrades as a result of exposure to UV and direct sunlight to form saluamine and other degradation products.[6, 11] Diffused daylight and fluorescent light does not cause this effect.[9] Storage of frusemide 1 mg/mL in sodium chloride 0.9% in burettes protected the solution from degradation due to direct sunlight.[11]

The stability of frusemide 2 mg/mL in glucose 5% and glucose 10% infusions was studied at room temperature under fluorescent lighting. No significant loss of frusemide was noted over a 24 hour period and no degradation products were detected. A minimal fall in pH occurred, and the number of particles present increased but stayed within BP limits. It was concluded that frusemide 2 mg/mL in glucose 5% and glucose 10% solution could be used over a 24 hour period but for no longer.[4]

Unpublished Information No change in appearance, pH or concentration was observed in an intravenous solution of frusemide 500 mg/300 mL (1.67 mg/mL) in glucose 5% over 41 hours at room temperature.[12]

Frusemide 40 mg or 80 mg in 50 mL sodium chloride 0.9% stored in two makes of PVC minibags was reported to be stable for three months at room temperature in the dark.[13]

Incompatibilities Frusemide injection has been reported to be physically or chemically incompatible with the following drug substances: amiodarone; amsacrine; benzylpenicillin; buprenorphine; chlorpromazine; ciprofloxacin; clarithromycin; diazepam; diltiazem; dobutamine; doxapram hydrochloride; doxorubicin hydrochloride; droperidol; erythromycin lactobionate; esmolol hydrochloride; filgrastim; fluconazole; gentamicin sulphate; idarubicin; isoprenaline hydrochloride; labetalol; metoclopramide; milrinone; netilmicin sulphate; ondansetron hydrochloride; papaveretum; pethidine hydrochloride; prochlorperazine; promethazine; quinidine; verapamil hydrochloride; vinblastine hydrochloride; vincristine hydrochloride; and vinorelbine tartrate.[14-18]

Compatibilities Frusemide 200 μg/mL and 400 μg/mL were studied in combination with hydrocortisone sodium succinate 300 μg/mL and 1 mg/mL in glucose 5% and sodium chloride 0.9% infusions using HPLC analysis. In each case, there was no more than 6% loss of frusemide after 24 hours at 25°C. For the higher strength hydrocortisone, there was 6-8% loss in 24 hours at 25°C but with the lower strength the loss was 10–14%.[10]

Frusemide 0.2 mg/mL with cefoperazone sodium 10 mg/mL in glucose 5% was studied at 4°C and 25°C, stored in the dark. Less than 5% degradation of both drugs occurred after two days at 25°C and five days at 4°C.[17]

Comments

In common clinical practice frusemide injection in sodium chloride 0.9% is stable for up to 28 days in conditions above pH 6.

References

1. ABPI. Compendium of data sheets and summaries of product characteristics 1996-1997. London: Datapharm Publications Ltd, 1996: 414-5.
2. Reynolds JEF, editor. Martindale: the extra pharmacopoeia, 31st edition. London: The Pharmaceutical Press, 1996: 870-3.
3. Crowe D. The stability of frusemide injection in polypropylene syringes. Pharm J 1992; 248: HS41.
4. Murdoch JM. Short term stability of frusemide 2 mg/mL in 5 per cent glucose and in 10 per cent glucose. Hosp Pharm Pract 1991; 1: 191-5.
5. Romankiewicz JA, et al. Medications not to be refrigerated. Am J Hosp Pharm 1979; 36: 1541-5.
6. Rowbotham PC, Stanford JB, Sugden JK. Some aspects of the photochemical degradation of frusemide. Pharm Acta Helv 1976; 51: 304-7.
7. Cruz JE, Maness DD, Yakatan GJ. Kinetics and mechanism of hydrolysis of furosemide. Int J Pharmaceutics 1979; 2: 275-81.
8. Connors KA, et al. Chemical stability of pharmaceuticals, 2nd edition. New York: John Wiley, 1986.
9. Neil JM, Fell AF, Smith G. Evaluation of the stability of frusemide in intravenous infusions by reversed-phase high-performance liquid chromatography. Int J Pharmaceutics 1984; 22: 105-26.
10. Stoberski P, Zakrzewski Z, Szulc A. Stability examination of furosemide and hydrocortisone sodium succinate by RP-HPLC in chosen infusion solution [in Polish]. Farm Pol 1988; 44: 398-401.
11. Yahya AM, McElnay JC, D'Arcy PF. Photodegradation of frusemide during storage in burette administration sets. Int J Pharmaceutics 1986; 31: 65-8.
12. Chandarana N. Personal communication, 1992.
13. Douch M, Bennett G. Personal communication, 1997.
14. Beatson C, Taylor A. A physical compatibility study of frusemide and flucloxacillin injections. Br J Pharm Pract 1987; 9: 223-6, 236.
15. Trissel LA. Handbook on injectable drugs, 9th edition. Bethesda, MD: American Society of Health-System Pharmacists Inc, 1996: 488-96.
16. Lund W, editor. The pharmaceutical codex: principles and practice of pharmaceutics, 12th edition. London: The Pharmaceutical Press, 1994: 875-9.
17. Lee DKT, Lee A, Wang D-P. Compatibility of cefoperazone sodium and furosemide in 5% dextrose injection. Am J Hosp Pharm 1991; 48: 108-10.
18. Taylor A. A physical compatibility study of clarithromycin injection with other commonly used injectable drugs. Pharm in Pract 1997; 7(9): 473-6.

Prepared by

Martin Callam

Ganciclovir

Approved Name
Ganciclovir

UK Proprietary Name
Cymevene (Roche Products Ltd)

Other Names
—

Product Details
Glass vials containing 546 mg of sterile, freeze-dried, ganciclovir powder equivalent to 500 mg of ganciclovir. The sodium content is approximately 2 mmol/500 mg. The reconstituted aqueous solution containing ganciclovir 50 mg/mL has a pH of 11.[1]

Preparation of Injection
The contents of each vial are reconstituted by dissolving in 10 mL of water for injection to give a solution of ganciclovir 50 mg/mL. If more accurate reconstitution is required (e.g. for paediatric use), the following powder displacement value may be used: 0.29 mL/500 mg.[2] Reconstituted vials should be inspected for particulate matter; if any is present the vial should be discarded. The required amount of ganciclovir solution should then be further diluted with typically 100 mL of: compound sodium lactate; glucose 5%; Ringer's solution; or sodium chloride 0.9%. Infusion solutions of a concentration greater than ganciclovir 10 mg/mL are not recommended.

Caution should be observed in the handling of ganciclovir and ingestion, inhalation, or direct contact with the skin or mucous membranes should be avoided. Ganciclovir should be considered a potential teratogen and carcinogen in humans.

Administration
Ganciclovir should be administered only by intravenous infusion, over at least one hour. Intramuscular or subcutaneous injection may result in severe tissue irritation.[1]

Vials distributed by the manufacturer prior to November 1995 required the infusion to be administered through a 5 µm in-line filter to remove any particulate matter, and are labelled with this instruction.

Stability in Practice
The manufacturer recommends that reconstituted vials are used immediately due to the possibility of crystal formation on storage and should not be refrigerated. Also, it is recommended that infusion solutions should be used within 24 hours of preparation to reduce the possibility of bacterial contamination. Infusion solutions may be refrigerated but should not be frozen.[1]

Published Information The stability of ganciclovir 1 mg/mL and 5 mg/mL, in glucose 5% and sodium chloride 0.9%, stored in PVC minibags for 35 days at 5°C and 25°C has been studied using HPLC analysis.[3] No significant loss of potency of any of the solutions studied was observed. A slight drop in pH occurred with both concentrations, in both infusions, but this did not exceed the manufacturers range of pH 9–11.

In a second study [4] concentrations of ganciclovir 1 mg/mL, 5 mg/mL, and 10 mg/mL showed a percentage drop in potency, confirmed by HPLC analysis, to 97.4%, 96.4%, and 93.4%, respectively, after 35 days storage. Again, no significant alteration in pH was noted.

The stability of ganciclovir 2 mg/mL and 4 mg/mL in 100 mL of sodium chloride 0.9% stored in PVC minibags has also been investigated.[5] Bags were stored at 4°C, protected from light, and samples analysed by HPLC at weekly intervals; bags were also inspected for visible particles. No ganciclovir degradation was detected after five weeks storage. Additionally, there was no reported change in pH and solutions remained free from particles.

Unpublished Information Ganciclovir 500 mg in 100 mL of sodium chloride 0.9% stored in a disposable elastomeric infusion device is said to be stable for five days at room temperature and 15 days when refrigerated.[6]

Ganciclovir 1–6 mg/mL, stored in either glucose 5% or sodium chloride 0.9%, is said to be stable in an infusion device for up to seven days at room temperature, 28 days at 6°C, and 63 days at -20°C.[7]

No loss of ganciclovir was detected by HPLC from 2 mg/mL or 4 mg/mL solutions in sodium chloride 0.9% stored in 100 mL PVC bags over 42 days at 5°C. A shelf-life of 21 days was suggested.[8]

Incompatibilities Ganciclovir sodium solution has been reported to be physically or chemically incompatible with the following drug substances: amifostine; amsacrine; aztreonam; cytarabine; doxorubicin hydrochloride; fludarabine phosphate; foscarnet sodium; ondansetron hydrochloride; piperacillin; piperacillin sodium-tazobactam sodium; sargramostim; and vinorelbine tartrate.[9,10] Ganciclovir sodium is also stated to be incompatible with solutions containing parahydroxybenzoates.[1]

Compatibilities Specialist references should be consulted for specific compatibility information.[8] Information on physical compatibility must be interpreted with care.

Comments

The available data suggest that ganciclovir (up to 10 mg/mL concentration) in glucose 5% or sodium chloride 0.9% stored in PVC minibags, is stable and compatible for up to 35 days at 5°C. In infusion devices, ganciclovir (up to 6 mg/mL concentration) in glucose 5% or sodium chloride 0.9%, may be stable for up to seven days at room temperature, 28 days at 6°C, and 63 days at -20°C.

References

1. ABPI. Compendium of data sheets and summaries of product characteristics 1996-1997. London: Datapharm Publications Ltd, 1996: 892-3.
2. Mulholland P. Displacement values of powder injections. Pharm J 1993; 251: 14-5.
3. Parasrampuria J, et al. Stability of ganciclovir sodium in 5% dextrose injection and in 0.9% sodium chloride injection over 35 days. Am J Hosp Pharm 1992; 49: 116-8.
4. Silvestri AP, et al. Stability and compatibility of ganciclovir sodium in 5% dextrose injection over 35 days. Am J Hosp Pharm 1991; 48: 2641-3.
5. Bennett G. The stability of ganciclovir in 0.9% sodium chloride injection. Pharm J 1992; 248(Suppl): HS41.
6. Fresenius Healthcare Group. Personal communication, 1992.
7. Baxter Healthcare Ltd. Personal communication, 1995.
8. Bennett G. Personal communication, 1994.
9. Trissel LA. Handbook on injectable drugs, 9th edition. Bethesda, MD: American Society of Health-System Pharmacists Inc, 1996: 499-501.
10. Trissel LA. Handbook on injectable drugs, 9th edition, supplement. Bethesda, MD: American Society of Health-System Pharmacists Inc, 1997: 50.

Prepared by

Charlotte Gibb and Duncan Petty

Gentamicin

Approved Name
Gentamicin sulphate

UK Proprietary Name
Cidomycin (Hoechst Marion Roussel Ltd)
Genticin (Roche Products Ltd)

Other Names
—

Product Details
The paediatric injection is available as 2 mL vials containing the equivalent of 20 mg of gentamicin base as the sulphate. The adult injection contains the equivalent of 80 mg of gentamicin base as the sulphate and is available as either 2 mL vials or ampoules. A 1 mL ampoule, containing the equivalent of 5 mg of gentamicin base as the sulphate is also available for intrathecal injection.[1,2] The BP injection has a pH of 3–5.[3]

An isotonic gentamicin infusion is also available (Baxter) containing 800 µg/mL of gentamicin as the sulphate in sodium chloride 0.9% in 100 mL PVC minibags.

The adult and paediatric injection, Cidomycin, contains methylhydroxybenzoate, propylhydroxybenzoate, and disodium edetate while the intrathecal injection contains sodium chloride.[1] Genticin is preservative free.[2]

The sodium content of Genticin is negligible. However, each available strength of Cidomycin contains 0.07 mmol/mL of sodium. The minibag presentation (Baxter) contains approximately 0.15 mmol/mL of sodium.

Preparation of Injection
The commercially available injections, and infusion are ready-to-use.

Administration
Gentamicin may be administered by either intramuscular or intravenous injection. If the intravenous route is used, gentamicin can be given as a bolus into the tubing of a 'giving set' or directly into the venous system over 2–3 minutes. Gentamicin may also be administered by intravenous infusion over no more than 20 minutes and in less than 100 mL of infusion fluid.[1]

Stability in Practice
Gentamicin sulphate is relatively stable with less than 10% degradation reported to have occurred in an injection stored for 2.5–3 years at 37°C.[4]

The commercially available injections should be stored at room temperature and not frozen.[1,2]

Published Information No loss of potency was reported for gentamicin 40 mg/mL injection diluted to a concentration of 10 mg/mL with sodium chloride 0.9% and stored in glass syringes at 4°C for 12 weeks.[5]

No degradation was observed by HPLC for an injection of gentamicin 10 mg/mL (as the sulphate) stored over a 14 day period in a two-piece polyethylene-polypropylene syringe at 2–8°C.[6]

Unpublished Information A paediatric injection containing gentamicin 10 mg/mL in 1 mL polypropylene syringes was found to be stable for at least seven days at room temperature. The rate of decomposition assessed by HPLC was reported to be 6% over a 12 day study period.[7]

The stability of gentamicin 0.8 mg/mL injection in an elastomeric infusion device has been reported to be 24 hours in sodium chloride 0.9% at room temperature or 30 days frozen (-20°C) for a 1 mg/mL solution. Gentamicin 0.6 mg/mL in glucose 5% is said to be stable for 30 days in a refrigerator and for a 1 mg/mL solution 30 days frozen at -20°C.[8]

Incompatibilities Gentamicin sulphate has been reported to be chemically or physically incompatible with the following drug substances: amphotericin B; carbenicillin; cephalosporins; cytarabine; erythromycin; frusemide; heparin; penicillins; sodium bicarbonate; and some TPN solutions.[1-4]

due to CO₂ liberation →gas/ dissolved

Compatibilities Gentamicin sulphate is compatible with the following infusion fluids: glucose 5%; Ringer's solution; and sodium chloride 0.9%.

Gentamicin sulphate 8 mg/L has been reported to be stable for eight hours at 37°C (simulated clinical conditions) when combined with azlocillin 500 mg/L stored in 1 L of peritoneal dialysis fluid containing glucose 1.36%.[9]

Gentamicin sulphate 8 mg/L has similarly been reported to be stable for 48 hours when stored at 4–37°C either alone or combined with cephazolin 75 mg/L and 150 mg/L in 1 L bags of peritoneal dialysis fluid containing glucose 1.5% and heparin 1000 units/L.[10]

Comments

In common clinical practice, gentamicin infusions are stable for at least seven days in sodium chloride 0.9% or glucose 5% at room temperature.

References

1. APBI. Compendium of data sheets and summaries of product characteristics 1996-1997. London: Datapharm Publications Ltd, 1996: 933-4.
2. ABPI. Compendium of data sheets and summaries of product characteristics 1996-1997. London: Datapharm Publications Ltd, 1996: 895-6.
3. Reynolds JEF, editor. Martindale: the extra pharmacopoeia, 31st edition. London: The Pharmaceutical Press, 1996: 235-8.
4. Lund W, editor. The pharmaceutical codex: principles and practice of pharmaceutics, 12th edition. London: The Pharmaceutical Press, 1994: 879-82.
5. Nahata MC, Hipple TF, Strausbaugh SD. Stability of gentamicin diluted in 0.9% sodium chloride injection in glass syringes. Hosp Pharm 1987; 22: 1131-2.
6. Parkinson R, et al. The stability of drugs in pre-filled syringes. Hosp Pharm Pract 1991; 1: 243-52.
7. Grassby P. Personal communication, 1996.
8. Fresenius Healthcare Group. Personal communication, 1996.
9. Roberts DE, et al. Azlocillin-aminoglycoside combinations in CAPD fluid. Br J Pharm Pract 1987; 9: 98-9.
10. Walker PC, Kaufmann RE, Massoud N. Compatibility of cefazolin and gentamicin in peritoneal dialysis solutions. Drug Intell Clin Pharm 1986; 20: 697-700.

Prepared by

James Thom

Heparin

Approved Name
Heparin calcium; heparin sodium.

UK Proprietary Name
See below.

Other Names
Soluble heparin (heparin sodium).

Product Details
A number of heparin calcium and heparin sodium preparations, in sodium chloride 0.9% and water for injection, are commercially available, with and without preservatives, and current compendia should be consulted for full product details.[1,2]

A 1% solution of either heparin calcium or heparin sodium has a pH of 5.5–8.0.[3]

Preparation of Injection
Most heparin preparations are ready-to-use or may be further diluted with glucose 5% or sodium chloride 0.9%. Care must be taken to ensure adequate mixing after additions of heparin, as the viscosity of heparin injections is such that 'pooling' may occur.

Administration
Heparin may be administered as an intravenous injection (bolus or infusion), or by subcutaneous infusion. Intramuscular injection is not recommended.

Stability in Practice
Heparin solutions may vary in colour from colourless to a pale straw colour. Minor colour variations do not indicate loss of potency. In aqueous solution, heparin stability is markedly reduced below pH 5.[3]

Commercially available preparations should be stored below 25°C protected from light, and from freezing.

Published Information Heparin preparations (1 unit/mL) in sodium chloride 0.9%, sterilised by autoclaving and stored at room temperature in daylight, have been reported to be stable for 12 months.[4] Heparin sodium 20 units/mL and 40 units/mL was found to be stable in sodium chloride 0.9%

at room temperature for 48 hours.[5] Several commercially available ampoules of heparin in sodium chloride 0.9% have shelf-lives of 24 months.

Opinion varies as to the stability of heparin in glucose intravenous infusions. Some workers suggest that rapid inactivation occurs[6] whereas others assert that there is no detectable loss in activity for up to 48 hours.[4,7,8] One reason that has been proposed for the loss of activity of heparin, is the acidity of commercial glucose solutions. However, in a number of studies, pH differences between heparin in glucose 5%, or in sodium chloride 0.9%, were minimal casting some doubt on this theory.[6,9,10]

Heparin sodium 1 unit/mL in glucose 3.75% with sodium chloride 0.225%, has been reported to be stable in 500 mL bags at room temperature (20–25°C) for 12 months. Samples stored in sodium chloride 0.9%, or glucose 2.5% with sodium chloride 0.9%, were also stable whilst heparin in glucose 5%, under the same storage conditions, was described as unstable although results indicated satisfactory potency was retained for up to seven days.[9]

The stability of heparin sodium 500 units/mL in 50 mL polypropylene syringes was investigated at room temperature and refrigerated (0–4°C). A gradual 8% loss of activity was noted after 21 days.[11]

At a concentration of 1 unit/mL in two-piece polyethylene/polypropylene syringes, no loss of heparin activity was observed over 52 weeks at 37°C. However, in polypropylene syringes with rubber-tipped plungers, extra peaks were noted in the UV spectrum, thought to be due to leaching of components from the rubber.[12]

The stability of heparin sodium 1000 units/mL and 40000 units/mL in polypropylene syringes designed for a portable pump-device was investigated by HPLC. Less than 3% loss of heparin sodium was observed over 30 days at 30°C.[13]

Incompatibilities Heparin calcium or sodium has been reported to be chemically or physically incompatible with the following drug substances: alteplase; amikacin sulphate; amiodarone; ampicillin; aprotinin; benzylpenicillin; cephalothin; chlorpromazine hydrochloride; ciprofloxacin; cytarabine; dacarbazine; daunorubicin; diazepam; dobutamine; doxorubicin; droperidol; erythromycin; gentamicin; haloperidol; hyaluronidase; hydrocortisone sodium succinate; kanamycin; labetalol hydrochloride; meperidine hydrochloride; methicillin; methotrimeprazine; netilmicin; opioid analgesics; oxytetracycline; polymixin B sulphate; promethazine hydrochloride; quinidine gluconate; streptomycin; tobramycin sulphate; triflupromazine hydrochloride; vancomycin; and vinblastine.[3,14,15]

Heparin is sometimes added to parenteral nutrition solutions, for which compatibility and maintenance of activity has been presumed from the absence of physical changes or loss of therapeutic effect. However, in the presence of calcium ions and fat emulsions, slow flocculation occurs. This may be due in part, to the formation of cross-links or bridges between the lipid droplets and the heparin molecules. The process may lead to extensive 'creaming' or separation in the parenteral nutrition mixture.[16]

Compatibilities The activity of heparin 35 units/mL in peritoneal dialysis fluids containing glucose 1.5% and 2.5% was investigated at 25°C and 4°C. Although a dip and recovery in activity was recorded between four and six hours at 25°C, activity was then retained for 14 days at 4°C.[17]

The compatibility of heparin sodium with teicoplanin in Hickman line catheters was investigated. Heparin 10 units/mL or 100 units/mL in sodium chloride 0.9% was mixed in equal quantity with teicoplanin 133 mg/mL. The resultant solution was instilled into a Hickman line catheter. No loss of activity of either drug was observed at 25°C for 24 hours. An 11% increase of teicoplanin was noted and attributed to the sorption of water by the silicone material of the catheter. Studies with heparin 20 units/mL or 40 units/mL in glucose 5% or sodium chloride 0.9% in glass flasks, found no significant changes or drug loss over 24 hours at 25°C.[18]

Comments

Heparin exhibits good aqueous stability in sodium chloride 0.9%, but the shelf-life appears to be limited in glucose solutions.

References

1. Mehta DK, editor. British national formulary, number 33. London: British Medical Association and the Royal Pharmaceutical Society of Great Britain, 1997: 105-7.
2. ABPI. Compendium of data sheets and summaries of product characteristics 1996-1997. London: Datapharm Publications Ltd, 1996.
3. Lund W, editor. The pharmaceutical codex: principles and practice of pharmaceutics, 12th edition. London: The Pharmaceutical Press, 1994: 895-7.
4. Bowie HM, Haylor V. Stability of heparin in sodium chloride solution. J Clin Pharm 1978; 3: 211-4.
5. Mitchell JF, Barger RC, Cantwell L. Heparin stability in 5% dextrose and 0.9% sodium chloride solutions. Am J Hosp Pharm 1976; 33: 540-2.
6. Pritchard J. Stability of heparin solutions. J Pharm Pharmacol 1964; 16: 487-9.
7. Moyle RS, Cain MJ. Observed stability of heparin in dextrose 5%. Aust J Hosp Pharm 1983; 13(3): 124.
8. Joy RT, et al. Effect of pH on the stability of heparin in 5% dextrose solutions. Am J Hosp Pharm 1979; 36: 618-21.
9. Wright A, Hecker J. Long term stability of heparin in dextrose-saline intravenous fluids. Int J Pharm Pract 1995; 3: 253-5.
10. Parker EA. Solution additive chemical incompatibility study. Am J Hosp Pharm 1967; 24: 434-9.
11. Tunbridge LJ, et al. Stability of diluted heparin stored in plastic syringes. Am J Hosp Pharm 1981; 38: 1001-4.
12. Parkinson R, et al. Stability of low-dose heparin in prefilled syringes. Br J Hosp Pharm Pract 1989; 11: 34, 36.
13. Stiles ML, Allen LV, McLaurey H-J. Stability of two concentrations of heparin sodium prefilled in CADD-Micro pump syringes. Int J Pharm Compounding 1997; 1: 433-4.
14. Reynolds JEF, editor. Martindale: the extra pharmacopoeia, 31st edition. London: The Pharmaceutical Press, 1996: 879-83.
15. Trissel LA. Handbook on injectable drugs, 9th edition. Bethesda, MD: American Society of Health-System Pharmacists Inc, 1996: 526-54.
16. Johnson OL, et al. The destabilisation of parenteral feeding emulsions by heparin. Int J Pharmaceutics 1989; 53: 237-40.
17. Matthews H. Heparin anticoagulant activity in intravenous fluids utilising a chromogenic substrate assay method. Aust J Hosp Pharm 1982; 12: S17-S22.
18. Malcomson C, et al. Investigations into the compatibility of teicoplanin with heparin. Eur J Parenter Sci 1997; 2: 51-5.

Prepared by

Tim Sizer and James Thom

Hydrocortisone Sodium Succinate

Approved Name

Hydrocortisone sodium succinate

UK Proprietary Name

Solu-Cortef (Pharmacia & Upjohn Ltd)

Other Names

—

Product Details

Glass vials containing a white, freeze-dried powder for reconstitution with water for injection. Each vial contains hydrocortisone sodium succinate equivalent to 100 mg of hydrocortisone. The product also contains sodium biphosphate and sodium phosphate.[1] Sodium content is approximately 0.21 mmol/vial.

Preparation of Injection

Reconstitute the contents of the vial with not more than 2 mL of water for injection and shake to dissolve. The pH of the reconstituted injection is pH 7–8.

Administration

Hydrocortisone sodium succinate may be administered by intramuscular injection, or intravenous bolus injection over 1–10 minutes. It may also be administered by intravenous infusion. A vial should be reconstituted with up to 2 mL water for injection which should then be added to 100–1000 mL (but not less than 100 mL) of glucose 5% or sodium chloride 0.9% infusion.

Stability in Practice

Vials should be stored at room temperature (15–30°C). In aqueous solution, over a wide pH range, hydrocortisone degrades by both oxidative and non-oxidative reactions of the C-17 dihydroxyacetone side chain.[2]

Spectrophotometric and microscopic investigation of the stability of hydrocortisone sodium succinate in glucose 5% and glucose 10% injections revealed the formation of crystals of hydrocortisone succinate during storage. The extent of crystallisation is dependent on the pH of the glucose solutions and length of storage.[3] Maximum stability occurs at pH 7–8.[3]

Published Information The manufacturer states that reconstituted solutions should be used immediately, and no diluents other than those recommended should be used.[1] Reconstituted injections should be inspected visually for particulate matter and discoloration prior to administration.

Hydrocortisone sodium succinate 0.1% solution in minibags is reported to have a shelf-life of three days at 25°C, or 26 days at 4°C in sodium chloride 0.9%; or 56 days at 4°C in glucose 5%.[4]

A 5% aqueous solution of hydrocortisone sodium succinate in polypropylene syringes was shown to have a shelf-life of three days at 25°C and 40 days at 4°C when protected from light.[4]

Unpublished Information Reconstituted solutions containing up to 1 mg/mL or greater than 25 mg/mL of hydrocortisone sodium succinate are said to be stable for up to 24 hours. Solutions between 1–25 mg/mL concentration are stable for only six hours due to the formation of micelles.[5]

Incompatibilities Hydrocortisone sodium succinate has been reported to be chemically or physically incompatible with the following drug substances: amylobarbitone sodium; chloramphenicol sodium succinate; ciprofloxacin; colistin sulphomethate sodium; dacarbazine; diazepam; doxapram hydrochloride; doxorubicin hydrochloride; ephedrine sulphate; heparin; hydralazine hydrochloride; kanamycin sulphate; metaraminol tartrate; midazolam hydrochloride; phenobarbitone sodium; prochlorperazine; tetracycline hydrochloride; and vancomycin hydrochloride.[2,3]

Compatibilities Specialist references should be consulted for specific compatibility information.[3]

Comments

The sodium content of hydrocortisone sodium succinate, when reconstituted with water, is 4.7 mg/mL.

Hydrocortisone sodium phosphate (Efcortesol) is also commercially available for parenteral use.[6]

References

1. ABPI. Compendium of data sheets and summaries of product characteristics 1996-1997. London: Datapharm Publications Ltd, 1996: 812-3.
2. Lund W, editor: The pharmaceutical codex: principles and practice of pharmaceutics, 12th edition. London: The Pharmaceutical Press, 1994: 901-7.
3. Trissel LA. Handbook on injectable drugs, 9th edition. Bethesda, MD: American Society of Health-System Pharmacists Inc, 1996: 562-78.
4. Small DC. The stability of reconstituted hydrocortisone sodium succinate injection in syringes and minibags. Pharm J 1992; 248: HS41.
5. Pharmacia & Upjohn Ltd. Personal communication, 1996.
6. ABPI. Compendium of data sheets and summaries of product characteristics 1996-1997. London: Datapharm Publications Ltd, 1996: 391-2.

Prepared by

Martin Lee

Imipenem with Cilastatin

Approved Name
Imipenem with Cilastatin

UK Proprietary Name
Primaxin (Merck Sharp & Dohme Ltd)

Other Names
Imipenem-cilastatin.

Product Details
Glass vials containing sterile powders of imipenem 250 mg (as the monohydrate) with cilastatin 250 mg (as the sodium salt) and glass vials containing imipenem 500 mg with cilastatin 500 mg. A monovial presentation is also available with a transfer needle attached to the vial containing imipenem 500 mg and cilastatin 500 mg. Primaxin does not contain aluminium, magnesium, or potassium ions.

The pH of the injection is 6.5–7.5.[1] Sodium content is approximately 0.86 mmol/250 mg vial, and 1.72 mmol/500 mg vial.[2] The osmolality of Primaxin 250 mg in water is 26 mosmol/mL; the osmolality of Primaxin 500 mg in 100 mL of water is 53 mosmol/mL.[2]

Preparation of Injection
The powder is reconstituted with either glucose 5% or sodium chloride 0.9% to a concentration of not less than 5 mg/mL. The monovial is reconstituted with infusion solution using the transfer needle, to a concentration of not less than 5 mg/mL.

The displacement value is 0.85% (100 mL added to 500 mg will give a volume of 100.85 mL).

Administration
Up to 500 mg (as imipenem) may be infused over 20–30 minutes. Doses of 1000 mg should be infused over 40–60 minutes.

Stability in Practice
Imipenem with cilastatin decomposes by hydrolysis with loss of antimicrobial activity due to cleavage of the beta-lactam ring.[3] Imipenem is unstable at acidic or alkaline pH; maximum stability of imipenem with cilastatin solution occurs at pH 6.5–7.5. The injection should be protected from light.

Published Information The manufacturer states that once reconstituted, solutions are stable for three hours at room temperature and 24 hours at 4°C.[4] Solutions that darken from a yellow colour to a brown colour indicate loss of potency.

Imipenem with cilastatin has been reported to be stable for 10 hours at room temperature when reconstituted with sodium chloride 0.9% and 48 hours at 4°C. The presence of sodium chloride 0.9% increases the stability while glucose decreases the stability and enhances decomposition. A loss of 15% of potency has been observed at -20°C and 10°C.[3]

Studies of imipenem with cilastatin sodium in various combinations of intravenous fluids produced the following stability data:[5]

Diluent	Stability at 4°C (hours)	Stability at 25°C (hours)
Glucose 5%	24	4
Glucose 10%	24	4
Glucose 5% with potassium chloride 0.15%	24	4
Glucose 5% with sodium chloride 0.225%	24	4
Glucose 5% with sodium chloride 0.9%	24	4
Mannitol 2.5%, 5% or 10%	24	4
Sodium chloride 0.9%	48	10

Incompatibilities Imipenem with cilastatin is incompatible with lactate. The manufacturer recommends that imipenem with cilastatin should not be mixed with other antibiotics.[4] Imipenem with cilastatin has been reported to be incompatible with the following drug substances: lorazepam; and midazolam hydrochloride.[6]

Compatibilities Imipenem with cilastatin is reported to be compatible with the following infusion fluids: glucose 5%; glucose 5% with sodium chloride 0.9%; glucose 5% with sodium chloride 0.225%; mannitol 2.5%; mannitol 5%; and sodium chloride 0.9%.[4]

Comments

Imipenem with cilastatin is reported to be chemically stable for at least 24 hours at 4°C when reconstituted with glucose 5% or sodium chloride 0.9%.

References

1. Reynolds JEF, editor. Martindale: the extra pharmacopoeia, 31st edition. London: The Pharmaceutical Press, 1996: 239-40.
2. Merck Sharp & Dohme Ltd. Personal communication, 1997.
3. Trissel LA. Handbook on injectable drugs, 9th edition. Bethesda, MD: American Society of Health-System Pharmacists Inc, 1996: 597-602.
4. ABPI. Compendium of data sheets and summaries of product characteristics 1996-1997. London: Datapharm Publications Ltd, 1996: 624-6.
5. Bigley FP, Forsyth RJ, Henley MW. Compatability of imipenem-cilastatin sodium with commonly used intravenous solutions. Am J Hosp Pharm 1986; 43: 2803-9.
6. Trissel LA. Handbook on injectable drugs, 9th edition, supplement. Bethesda, MD: American Society of Health-System Pharmacists Inc, 1997: 60.

Prepared by

Krissy Cock

Meropenem

Approved Name

Meropenem

UK Proprietary Name

Meronem (Zeneca)

Other Names

Merrem.

Product Details

Glass vials containing the equivalent of 250 mg, 500 mg, or 1 g of meropenem. The injection consists of a sterile powder containing meropenem as the tri-hydrate, blended with anhydrous sodium carbonate (meropenem 1 g contains 3.9 mmol of sodium).

Preparation of Injection

The content of each vial is reconstituted by the addition of 4.78 mL of water for injection for each 250 mg of meropenem to give a solution containing meropenem 50 mg/mL. The pH of a solution reconstituted with water for injection is 7.7.

Meropenem may also be directly reconstituted with a compatible infusion fluid and then further diluted (50–200 mL) with the infusion fluid as required. Meropenem may be diluted (1–20 mg/mL) with the following solutions: glucose 5%; glucose 10%; glucose 5% with potassium chloride 0.15%; glucose 5% with sodium bicarbonate 0.02%; glucose 5% with sodium chloride 0.225%; glucose 5% with sodium chloride 0.9%; mannitol 2.5%; mannitol 10%; and sodium chloride 0.9%.

The displacement value for meropenem is 0.22 mL/250 mg.

Administration

Meropenem 250 mg/5 mL in water for injection may be administered as an intravenous bolus injection over five minutes or as an intravenous infusion (50–200 mL) over 15–30 minutes.

Stability in Practice

The manufacturer states that freshly prepared solutions should be used whenever possible and that the reconstituted injection containing meropenem 1–20 mg/mL should be used immediately and must be stored for no longer than 24 hours, under refrigeration, only if necessary.[1] However, reconstituted solutions of meropenem are said to maintain satisfactory potency at room temperature (15–25°C) or under refrigeration (4°C) for the periods shown below:

Diluent	Stability at 4°C (hours)	Stability at 25°C (hours)
Glucose 5%	14	3
Glucose 10%	8	2
Glucose 5% with potassium chloride 0.15%	14	3
Glucose 5% with sodium bicarbonate 0.02%	8	2
Glucose 5% with sodium chloride 0.225%	14	3
Glucose 5% with sodium chloride 0.9%	14	3
Mannitol 2.5% or 10%	14	3
Sodium chloride 0.9%	48	8

Published Information The chemical stability of meropenem has been investigated as an aqueous solution of equimolar amounts of meropenem and sodium hydrogen carbonate. Analysis was by HPLC assay, with a drug concentration of 400 mg/mL. Storage was at 30°C for up to 24 hours; details of light protection were not indicated. HPLC analysis suggested the major degradation product to be a beta-lactam hydrolysed product and the minor degradation product to be a dimer. Other degradation products were only present in trace amounts. The dimer was believed to exist as a mixture of double-bonded isomers, the proportion of which varied with pH. Even at high concentration, the time required to reach 90% of initial potency was about 15 hours at pH 7 and about 11 hours at pH 8.[2,3]

The stability of meropenem in a variety of infusion fluids was investigated in PVC bags, glass vials, and in the ADD-Vantage System (Abbott), or Minibag Plus System (Baxter). The nature of the infusion fluid influenced the stability. HPLC results indicated that meropenem 1 mg/mL or 20 mg/mL in PVC bags in sodium chloride 0.9% or water for injection was stable for at least 48 hours at 4–5°C or 21–26°C. The same dilutions in glucose 5% were stable for four hours at 21–26°C or 16 hours at 4–5°C.[4]

In glass vials and the ADD-Vantage System or Minibag Plus System meropenem 2.5 mg/mL or 50 mg/mL was stable in sodium chloride 0.9% or water for injection for up to 48 hours at 4–5°C or 21–26°C. In glucose 5%, a shelf-life of up to 48 hours was also indicated.[4]

Unpublished Information   The chemical stability of meropenem 1 g/20 mL in water for injection stored in 20 mL plastic syringes has been investigated by HPLC. Storage was at 4–8°C for four days.[5] Results indicated a 4% loss of meropenem per day suggesting a shelf-life of 24 hours at 4°C.

Compatibilities   Compatibility has been demonstrated with the following intravenous solutions: compound sodium lactate; glucose 5%; glucose 10%; glucose 5% with potassium chloride 0.15%; glucose 5% with sodium bicarbonate 0.02%; glucose 5% with sodium chloride 0.2%; glucose 5% with sodium chloride 0.9%; mannitol 2.5%; mannitol 10%; Ringer's solution; sodium chloride 0.45%; sodium chloride 0.9%; and sodium lactate N/6 solution.[4]

Comments

In common clinical practice, meropenem is stable for up to 24 hours in glucose 5% and sodium chloride 0.9% at room temperature.

References

1. ABPI. Compendium of data sheets and summaries of product characteristics 1996-1997. London: Datapharm Publications Ltd, 1996: 1291-3.
2. Takeuchi Y, et al. The stability of a novel carbapenem antibiotic, meropenem (SM-7338), in a solid state formulation for injection. Chem Pharm Bull (Tokyo) 1993; 41(11): 1998-2002.
3. Takeuchi Y, et al. Stability of a 1ß-methylcarbapenem antibiotic, meropenem (SM-7338) in aqueous solution. Chem Pharm Bull (Tokyo) 1995; 43(4): 689-92.
4. Patel PR, Cook SE. Stability of meropenem in intravenous solutions. Am J Health-Syst Pharm 1997; 54: 412-21.
5. Whicker S. Personal communication, 1996.

Prepared by

Brian Baker and Christine Trehane

Metoclopramide

Approved Name
Metoclopramide hydrochloride

UK Proprietary Name
Maxolon (Monmouth Pharmaceuticals)

Maxolon High Dose (Monmouth Pharmaceuticals)

A non-proprietary 10mg/2mL injection and a 100mg/20mL injection is also commercially available.

Other Names
—

Product Details
Each 2mL ampoule of metoclopramide injection contains metoclopramide hydrochloride 5mg/mL. The product also contains sodium chloride and sodium metabisulphite. The pH is between 3–5 and the osmolality is 280mosmol/kg.

High dose metoclopramide (Maxolon High Dose) is only licensed for use with cytotoxic chemotherapy. Each 20mL ampoule contains metoclopramide hydrochloride 5 mg/mL, and contains sodium chloride. The pH is 5–6.5.

Sodium content is approximately 0.27mmol for the 10mg/2mL injection, and 2.74mmol for the 100mg/20mL injection.

Preparation of Injection
The injection is presented in a ready-to-use form.

Administration
Metoclopramide may be administered by intramuscular injection, or by slow intravenous injection over 1–2 minutes. High doses may be administered intravenously by infusion after dilution with glucose 5% or sodium chloride 0.9%.

The preferred method of administration is as a continuous infusion with a loading dose given in 50–100mL of diluent over 15–20 minutes. A maintenance dose diluted with 500mL of diluent may be given over 8–12 hours, or intermittent infusion used with the dose diluted with at least 50mL of diluent and given at least 15 minutes before starting chemotherapy.

Stability in Practice
Metoclopramide undergoes hydrolysis with the formation of 2-diethylaminoethylamine and other decomposition products.[1] Solutions become discoloured following exposure to light.

Solutions of metoclopramide for injection are reported to be stable within the range pH 2–9. The injection should be protected from light and stored in a cool place, in its original carton. Ampoules showing signs of discoloration should be discarded.

Published Information   Metoclopramide is physically compatible with compound sodium lactate, glucose 5%, and sodium chloride 0.9%, and is stable for 48 hours provided solutions are protected from light, or 24 hours when not protected from light.[2]

Metoclopramide 5mg/mL in polypropylene syringes was stable for at least 90 days at 4°C, 60 days at 23°C, and seven days at 32°C. Stability being defined as the retention of more than 90% of initial metoclopramide concentration. Freezing the solution caused unacceptable precipitation.[3]

Physical compatibility with diamorphine, for up to 96 hours, has been reported but some discoloration was noted.[4]

Unpublished Information   Metoclopramide 400mg/100mL in sodium chloride 0.9% stored in PVC bags is said to undergo 9% decomposition after seven days at 4°C and 10% at 20°C.

In polypropylene syringes, metoclopramide 10mg/2mL is said to have shown no sign of decomposition when stored at 4°C and 20°C for 35 days.[5]

Metoclopramide 10mg/2mL is said to be compatible with morphine 10mg, and with diamorphine 100mg, both for six days at room temperature. Compatibility is not satisfactory between metoclopramide 10mg and morphine 100mg due to poor solubility.[6]

High dose metoclopramide is said to be stable for 48 hours at room temperature with morphine hydrochloride 100mg or diamorphine hydrochloride 50mg when diluted 1 in 10 with sodium chloride 0.9%.[6]

Metoclopramide is also said to be stable with pethidine at 10:100 and 100:100 level for six days at room temperature when protected from light.

Incompatibilities   Metoclopramide hydrochloride

solutions have been reported to be incompatible with the following drug substances: allopurinol; amphotericin B; amsacrine; cephalothin sodium; chloramphenicol sodium succinate; diazepam; flucloxacillin; phenytoin; and sodium bicarbonate. Possible incompatibility has also been reported with: ampicillin sodium; benzylpenicillin potassium; calcium gluconate; cisplatin; cyclizine; erythromycin lactobionate; frusemide; lorazepam; methotrexate sodium; and tetracycline hydrochloride.[2,7]

Compatibilities High dose metoclopramide (Maxolon High Dose) is stated by the manufacturers to be compatible with cisplatin, cyclophosphamide, and doxorubicin hydrochloride over specified concentration ranges and is stable for 24 hours at room temperature when protected from light. Metoclopramide is also reported to be compatible with morphine and diamorphine over specified concentration ranges for 48 hours at room temperature under normal fluorescent light.[8]

The stability of a mixture of morphine sulphate 1 mg/mL and metoclopramide hydrochloride 0.5 mg/mL in glucose 5% or sodium chloride 0.9% contained in infusion devices, syringes, and PVC bags was investigated. The results demonstrated that the stability was related to the metoclopramide component and was dependent on the diluent used. Metoclopramide was reported to be more stable in sodium chloride 0.9% than in glucose 5%.[9]

Comments

Care should be taken when interpreting stability data due to possible differences in formulations.

References

1. Lund W, editor. The pharmaceutical codex: principles and practice of pharmaceutics, 12th edition. London: The Pharmaceutical Press, 1994: 956-8.
2. Trissel LA. Handbook on injectable drugs, 9th edition. Bethesda, MD: American Society of Health-System Pharmacists Inc, 1996: 721-32.
3. Zhang Y, et al. Stability of metoclopramide hydrochloride in plastic syringes. Am J Health-Syst Pharm 1996; 53: 1300-2.
4. Rogers GC, Davies MB, Allwood MC. An investigation into the stability of diamorphine hydrochloride with diazepam, metoclopramide or methotrimeprazine. Int Pharm J 1991; 5: 70.
5. Haines-Nutt F. Personal communication, 1996.
6. Monmouth Pharmaceuticals. Personal communication, 1996.
7. Reynolds JEF, editor. Martindale: the extra pharmacopoeia, 31st edition. London: The Pharmaceutical Press, 1996: 1228-30.
8. ABPI. Compendium of data sheets and summaries of product characteristics 1996-1997. London: Datapharm Publications Ltd, 1996: 639-41.
9. Nixon AR, O'Hare MCB, Chisakuta AM. The stability of morphine sulphate and metoclopramide hydrochloride in various delivery presentations. Pharm J 1995; 254: 153-5.

Prepared by

Martin Lee

Metronidazole

Approved Name

Metronidazole

UK Proprietary Name

Flagyl (Rhône-Poulenc Rorer Ltd)
Metrolyl (Lagap Pharmaceuticals Ltd)
Non-proprietary preparations are also available.

Other Names

—

Product Details

Metronidazole 5 mg/mL is available as a colourless solution in 100 mL bottles, 100 mL bags, or 20 mL ampoules. The injection also contains sodium phosphate, citric acid, and sodium chloride. The ready-to-use injection has a pH of 5–7 and an osmolality of 310 mosmol/kg.[1,2]

Sodium content is 13.6 mmol/100 mL (Flagyl), and 14.53 mmol/100 mL (Metrolyl).

Preparation of Injection

No further dilution is required.

Administration

Metronidazole should be administered by intermittent intravenous infusion over 20–30 minutes, with a maximum infusion rate of 5 mL/hour.

Stability in Practice

Metronidazole solutions are clear and colourless, and should be stored between 15–30°C, protected from light. Whereas short-term exposure to normal room light does not adversely affect the stability, prolonged exposure will cause a darkening of the solution.

Maximum stability of metronidazole is at pH 5.6.[3]

Published Information Undiluted metronidazole 5 mg/mL, and metronidazole diluted with glucose 5% to a concentration of 1 mg/mL, was stable over a four month period, with no loss of activity, when stored in pre-filled syringes.[4]

Unpublished Information The stability of ce-furoxime 750 mg in metronidazole 5 mg/mL solution stored frozen in 100 mL bags has been investigated. No loss or breakdown of either drug was said to have occurred after six months. Once thawed, it is recommended that bags are used within three days. A precipitation, probably metronidazole, occurs but disappears once the solution reaches room temperature.[5]

Incompatibilities Metronidazole solutions have been reported to be physically or chemically incompatible with the following drug substances: amino acid solutions; ampicillin sodium; aztreonam; benzylpenicillin potassium; cephalothin sodium; cephamandole nafate; cefoxitin sodium; compound sodium lactate; dopamine hydrochloride; filgrastim; and glucose 10%.[1,2,6]

Compatibilities Cefuroxime sodium is physically and chemically compatible with metronidazole 5 mg/mL infusion. It is recommended that an admixture of 750 mg cefuroxime sodium in 100 mL of metronidazole 5 mg/mL may be assigned a shelf-life of seven days when stored at 4°C.[7]

Specialist reference sources should be consulted for further compatibility information.[1]

Comments

In common clinical practice, metronidazole solutions are used in their commercially available ready-to-use form, stored at room temperature away from direct sunlight, and therefore stability problems are not usually an issue. However, many CIVAS do add cefuroxime 750 mg or 1.5 g to metronidazole infusions to facilitate more convenient administration of this commonly used combination of antibiotics for surgical prophylaxis and treatment.

References

1. Trissel LA. Handbook on injectable drugs, 9th edition. Bethesda, MD: American Society of Health-System Pharmacists Inc, 1996: 733-9.
2. ABPI. Compendium of data sheets and summaries of product characteristics 1996-1997. London: Datapharm Publications Ltd, 1996: 856-7.
3. Wang D-P, Yeh M-K. Degradation kinetics of metronidazole in solution. J Pharm Sci 1993; 82: 95-8.
4. Parkinson R, et al. The stability of drugs in pre-filled syringes: gentamicin, benzylpenicillin and metronidazole. Hosp Pharm Pract 1991; 1: 243-54.

5. Midcalf B. Personal communication, 1996.

6. Reynolds JEF, editor. Martindale: the extra pharmacopoeia, 31st edition. London: The Pharmaceutical Press, 1996: 621-5.

7. Barnes AR. Chemical stabilities of cefuroxime sodium and metronidazole in an admixture for intravenous infusion. J Clin Pharm Ther 1990; 15: 187-96.

Prepared by

Suzanne Kendall-Smith

Morphine

Approved Name
Morphine sulphate

UK Proprietary Name
—

Other Names
Morphine sulfate.

Product Details
Clear glass ampoules containing 10, 15, 20, and 30mg/mL of morphine as the sulphate in 1mL and 2mL. Morphine is also available in 2mL Min-I-Jet (IMS) containing 10mg/2mL morphine sulphate. The pH of the injection is 2.5–6. Osmolality of a 10mg/mL injection (as the hydrochloride) is 54mosmol/kg.

Disposable syringes, Rapiject (IMS), containing morphine sulphate 50mg/mL and 100mg/mL are also available.

Preparations may contain sodium metabisulphite 0.1% as antioxidant.

Preparation of Injection
The injection is presented in a ready-to-use form.

Administration
Morphine is usually administered as the sulphate although the hydrochloride and tartrate are used in similar doses. The acetate has also been used.

A number of routes of administration can be used. When administered by subcutaneous or intramuscular injection, 10mg every four hours is usually used but doses may be between 5–20mg or greater.

With slow intravenous injection, up to 15mg is used which may be the loading dose for continuous or patient controlled infusion. For continuous intravenous or subcutaneous administration, 0.8–80mg per hour may be administered although some patients have required much higher doses.

With intraspinal injection, 5mg is given initially as an epidural injection. Further doses of 1–2mg may be given for adequate pain relief up to a total of 10mg in 24 hours. For continuous epidural infusion, 2–4mg per 24 hours, increased if necessary by 1–2mg is used.

Intrathecal injection is less common than epidural administration. A dose of 0.2–1mg on a single occasion has been used.[1]

Stability in Practice
Morphine is the principal alkaloid of opium used for the control of moderate to severe pain. Morphine salts are sensitive to changes in pH with a tendency to precipitate out of solution in an alkaline environment. Morphine sulphate darkens on prolonged exposure to light.

Morphine is oxidised by atmospheric oxygen to produce the dimer, pseudomorphine, and also morphine-*N*-oxide.[2] However, the degradation products do not differ greatly from morphine in their qualitative pharmacological effects and the loss of active ingredient is a more important consideration than the build up of degradation products.[3]

A shelf-life of one year for intrathecal morphine has been recommended.

Published Information A variety of studies have been performed to determine the stability of morphine sulphate stored in syringes.

Morphine sulphate 2mg/mL in sodium chloride 0.9% has been reported to be chemically stable for six weeks when stored in polypropylene syringes at room temperature, but a similar solution also containing sodium metabisulphite 0.1% lost 15% potency in the same period.[4] Stability of such solutions with or without antioxidant in glass syringes was considered unacceptable.[5]

A further study investigated the stability of morphine sulphate 1mg/mL and 5mg/mL in plastic syringes for use in patient controlled analgesia (PCA) devices, using HPLC. Data indicated that morphine was stable for at least six weeks when stored at -20°C, 4°C, and 23°C, protected from light, but only for about one week when stored at 23°C exposed to light.[6]

Solutions of morphine sulphate 2mg/mL and 15mg/mL were filled into a disposable glass syringe, PVC container, and two types of disposable infusion device. Stability was determined at room temperature and 4°C, and also at 31°C in the infusion devices. Morphine sulphate remained stable for at least 12 days in all of the containers and devices and at each temperature studied.[7]

Injectable solutions of morphine sulphate in concentrations ranging from 1–25 mg/mL were shown to be stable when stored at refrigerated temperature for 30 days in a prefilled CADD pump reservoir followed by 14 days at room temperature, and for at least 60 days (morphine hydrochloride) when stored at 32°C.[8,9] However, a rise in concentration may be expected due to evaporation of the vehicle during storage.

Morphine sulphate solutions at concentrations of 1 mg/mL or 2 mg/mL in glucose 5% and sodium chloride 0.9% have been reported to be stable for 14 weeks when frozen at -20°C in PVC bags.[10]

Morphine sulphate 1 mg/mL in bacteriostatic sodium chloride 0.9% (containing benzyl alcohol 1 mg/mL) stored in glass vials at 22°C and 4°C has been reported to be stable for 91 days.[11]

Unpublished Information Samples of morphine sulphate 1 mg/mL in glucose 5% and sodium chloride 0.9% stored in plastic syringes at 4°C, room temperature, and 35°C have been claimed to show no significant degradation after 90 days and 210 days.[12,13]

Morphine sulphate 2 mg/mL in a PCA infusion device in both glucose 5% and sodium chloride 0.9% has been claimed to be stable for 76 days.

Morphine sulphate 1–20 mg/mL in glucose 5% in an infusion device is said to have a shelf-life of 57 days at 2–8°C plus three days at room temperature, or 99 days at 2–8°C.[14] Morphine sulphate 1–15 mg/mL in glucose 5% is said to have a shelf-life of 102 days at room temperature.[14]

Incompatibilities Morphine sulphate has been reported to be incompatible with the following drug substances: aciclovir; aminophylline; barbiturates (sodium salts); chlorpromazine hydrochloride; flucloxacillin; fluorouracil; frusemide; heparin sodium (there is some evidence to show incompatibility at morphine concentrations greater than 5 mg/mL);[15] methicillin sodium; nitrofurantoin; pethidine hydrochloride; phenytoin sodium; prochlorperazine edisylate; promethazine hydrochloride; sodium bicarbonate; and tetracyclines.[1,16]

Compatibilities Specialist references should be consulted for specific compatibility information.[16]

Morphine and droperidol have been reported to be physically and chemically compatible at a wide range of concentrations, however data are variable. The combination of morphine sulphate 2 mg/mL with droperidol 0.2 mg/mL has been shown to be stable for 14 days at room temperature in plastic syringes.[17] In an unpublished study on morphine sulphate 2 mg/mL with droperidol 0.12 mg/mL a shelf-life of one month at 22°C (plus seven days at 32°C), and four months at 4°C for both syringe and elastomeric presentations has been claimed.[18] A further unpublished study suggested a shelf-life of 182 days at 4°C, or 35 days at 22°C (plus seven days at 32°C) for both presentations.[14]

Metoclopramide 0.5 mg/mL is reported to be more stable with sodium chloride 0.9% as diluent than with glucose 5% when combined with morphine 1 mg/mL. Such mixtures are said to be stable for about 14 days at 22°C and at least four months at 4°C in infusion devices, syringes, and bags.[14,19]

When admixed in sodium chloride 0.9% injection, ondansetron 0.1 mg/mL and 1 mg/mL plus morphine sulphate 1 mg/mL were compatible and stable for at least seven days at 32°C and at least 31 days at 4°C and 22°C in PVC containers.[20]

Morphine sulphate 0.02 mg/mL with bupivacaine hydrochloride 1 mg/mL in sodium chloride 0.9% stored in 100 mL bags is said to be stable for at least seven days when tested at temperatures from 4–60°C.[21]

Ketamine 1 mg/mL with morphine sulphate 20 mg/mL in sodium chloride 0.9% stored in plastic syringes has been reported to be stable for at least four days.[22]

Comments

Morphine sulphate in PVC bags and polypropylene syringes appears to be stable for at least six weeks at room temperature.

In CADD pump reservoirs morphine sulphate is stable for 30 days, if refrigerated, followed by 14 days at room temperature.

Stability in infusion devices in glucose 5% at 2–8°C is 57 days plus three days at room temperature.

References

1. Reynolds JEF, editor. Martindale: the extra pharmacopoeia, 31st edition. London: The Pharmaceutical Press, 1996: 63-7.
2. Yeh S-Y, Lach JL. Stability of morphine in aqueous solution III: kinetics of morphine degradation in aqueous solution. J Pharm Sci 1961; 50: 35-43.
3. Deeks T, Davis S, Nash S. Stability of an intrathecal morphine

injection formulation. Pharm J 1983; 230: 495-7.

4. Grassby PF. The stability of morphine sulphate in 0.9% sodium chloride stored in plastic syringes. Pharm J 1992; 248: HS24-HS25.

5. Grassby PF, Hutchings L. Factors affecting the physical and chemical stability of morphine sulphate solutions stored in syringes. Int J Pharm Pract 1993; 2: 39-43.

6. Strong ML, et al. Shelf-lives and factors affecting the stability of morphine sulphate and meperidine (pethidine) hydrochloride in plastic syringes for use in patient-controlled analgesic devices. J Clin Pharm Ther 1994; 19: 361-9.

7. Duafala ME, et al. Stability of morphine sulfate in infusion devices and containers for intravenous administration. Am J Hosp Pharm 1990; 47: 143-6.

8. Stiles ML, Tu Y-H, Allen LV. Stability of morphine sulfate in portable pump reservoirs during storage and simulated administration. Am J Hosp Pharm 1989; 46: 1404-7.

9. Roos PJ, et al. Stability of morphine hydrochloride in a portable pump reservoir. Pharm Weekbl (Sci) 1992; 14: 23-6.

10. Depiero D, et al. Stability of morphine sulphate solutions frozen in polyvinyl chloride intravenous bags. Pharm Pract News 1987; 14(Oct): 39-40.

11. Nahata MC, Morosco RS, Hipple TF. Stability of morphine sulfate in bacteriostatic 0.9% sodium chloride injection stored in glass vials at two temperatures. Am J Hosp Pharm 1992; 49: 2785-6.

12. Belmonte A, Bolton S. Personal communication, 1986.

13. Campbell A, Nixon A. Patient controlled analgesia (letter). Pharm J 1991; 247: 456.

14. Baxter Ltd. Personal communication, 1996.

15. Baker DE, et al. Compatibility of heparin sodium and morphine sulfate. Am J Hosp Pharm 1985; 42: 1352-5.

16. Trissel LA. Handbook on injectable drugs, 9th edition. Bethesda, MD: American Society of Health-System Pharmacists Inc, 1996: 761-72.

17. Williams OA, et al. Stability of morphine and droperidol, separately and combined, for use as an infusion. Hosp Pharm Pract 1992; 2: 597-600.

18. Belfast City Hospital. Personal communication, 1993.

19. Nixon AR, O'Hare MCB, Chisakuta AM. The stability of morphine sulphate and metoclopramide hydrochloride in various delivery presentations. Pharm J 1995; 254: 153-5.

20. Trissel LA, et al. Compatibility and stability of ondansetron hydrochloride with morphine sulfate and hydromorphone hydrochloride in 0.9% sodium chloride injection at 4, 22 and 32°C. Am J Hosp Pharm 1994; 51: 2138-42.

21. Storey R. Personal communication, 1996.

22. Middleton M, Edwards ND, Reilly CS. Do morphine and ketamine keep? Hosp Pharm Pract 1994; 4: 57-8.

Prepared by

Claire McIntyre

Ofloxacin

Approved Name

Ofloxacin

UK Proprietary Name

Tarivid (Hoechst Marion Roussel Ltd)

Other Names

—

Product Details

Clear glass vials containing ofloxacin (as the hydrochloride) in a clear greenish-yellow solution, with sodium chloride for isotonicity and hydrochloric acid to adjust to pH 4.5. Available in concentrations of 100 mg/50 mL, and 200 mg/100 mL.[1]

The injection has a pH of 3.5–5.5. A 0.4 mg/mL solution in sodium chloride 0.9% has an osmolality of 281 mosmol/kg, while a 0.4 mg/mL solution in glucose 5% has an osmolality of 259 mosmol/kg.[2]

Sodium content is 15.4 mmol/200 mg.

Note that 1.1 mg of ofloxacin hydrochloride is equivalent to 1 mg of ofloxacin.

Preparation of Injection

The injection is presented in a ready-to-use form.

Administration

Ofloxacin injection is normally administered undiluted, as an infusion, over not less than 30 minutes. Infusions should be prepared by aseptically diluting the injection with glucose 5% or sodium chloride 0.9%. Infusions are stable for 72 hours at room temperature.[2]

Stability in Practice

Ofloxacin is a flouroquinolone antibiotic with good aqueous stability in a variety of injectable diluents.[2,3] Ofloxacin is amphoteric, and poorly soluble at neutral pH; solubility increases at higher or lower pH.

The undiluted injection has a shelf-life of two years. Injections should be stored at room temperature (15–30°C) and protected from light. Brief exposure to temperatures above 40°C does not affect stability.

Diluted solutions in glucose 5% or sodium chloride 0.9% are stable for at least three days at 24°C or 14 days at 5°C.[2]

Colour intensity is not reflective of potency.

Published Information The stability of diluted ofloxacin infusion solutions has been investigated using degradation sensitive HPLC techniques.[2,3]

A variety of intravenous solutions containing ofloxacin 0.4 mg/mL and ofloxacin 4.0 mg/mL (as the hydrochloride) were stored in PVC minibags at 24°C for three days, 5°C for seven and 14 days, and at -20°C for 13 and 26 weeks followed by 14 days at 5°C. An assessment of ofloxacin degradation, pH, visual incompatibility and particulates showed that in all solutions tested, ofloxacin was stable at all storage conditions. However, in mannitol 20% crystals formed at 5°C and -20°C, probably due to salting-out effects.[2]

Glucose 5% or sodium chloride 0.9% intravenous solutions containing ofloxacin 0.8 mg/mL were stored in PVC minibags for simulated infusion over one hour, and for six hours at room temperature without light protection. No evidence of sorption or significant degradation of ofloxacin was noted.[3]

Ofloxacin is sensitive to UV light, losing potency if exposed to 1 J of irradiation per cm^3 UVA at a wavelength of 300–400 nm. The bi-products of photodegradation are reported to be toxic and may induce photosensitivity in some patients.[4]

Incompatibilities Ofloxacin solutions have been reported to be incompatible with the following drug substances: cefepime hydrochloride; and flucloxacillin sodium.[5,6]

Compatibilities Specialist references should be consulted for specific compatibility information.[6]

Ofloxacin hydrochloride injection is chemically and physically compatible with the following intravenous solutions: glucose 5%; glucose 5% with sodium chloride 0.9%; Ringer's solution; and sodium chloride 0.9%.[1,2]

Compatibility has been demonstrated, with little or no loss of either drug over 48 hours, as determined by an HPLC method, with the following intravenous antibiotic injections at a variety of concentrations and storage conditions: amoxycillin sodium; ceftazidime; clindamycin phosphate; gentamicin sulphate; piperacillin sodium; tobramycin sulphate; and vancomycin hydrochloride.[5]

Comments

Ofloxacin intravenous injection is a stable, isotonic injection normally administered undiluted. It may be added to intravenous infusion solutions such as glucose 5% or sodium chloride 0.9% without significant degradation occurring over 72 hours at room temperature. Co-administration with other drugs is best avoided, though compatibility with some antibiotics has been investigated.[5]

References

1. ABPI. Compendium of data sheets and summaries of product characteristics 1996-1997. London: Datapharm Publications Ltd, 1996: 422-3.

2. Bornstein M, et al. Stability of an ofloxacin injection in various infusion fluids. Am J Hosp Pharm 1992; 49: 2756-60.

3. Faouzi MA, et al. Stability and compatibility studies of pefloxacin, ofloxacin and ciprofloxacin with PVC infusion bags. Int J Pharmaceutics 1993; 89: 125-31.

4. Matsumoto M, et al. Photostability and biological activity of fluoroquinolones substituted at the 8 position after UV irradiation. Antimicrob Agents Chemother 1992; 36(8): 1715-9.

5. Janknegt R, et al. Ofloxacin intravenous compatibility with other antibacterial agents. Pharm Weekbl (Sci) 1991; 13: 207-9.

6. Trissel LA. Handbook on injectable drugs, 9th edition. Bethesda, MD: American Society of Health-System Pharmacists Inc, 1996: 817-9.

Prepared by

Tim Sizer

Pethidine

Approved Name
Pethidine hydrochloride

UK Proprietary Name
—

Other Names
Meperidine hydrochloride.

Product Details
Snap-break ampoules containing pethidine hydrochloride in preservative free water for injection. Strengths available include: 50 mg/mL; 100 mg/2 mL; 50 mg/5 mL; 100 mg/5 mL.

The injection has a pH of 3–5. The osmolality of a 50 mg/mL solution is 302 mosmol/kg.[1] The injection is sodium free.

Preparation of Injection
Ampoules are ready-to-use. The injection may be diluted with glucose 5% or sodium chloride 0.9%.

Administration
Pethidine may be administered by slow intravenous injection over 3–5 minutes; dilution with water for injection is advised. Continuous small volume infusion (10–50 mL) may also be used, using an accurately controlled syringe driver or similar device.

Infusions may be prepared with glucose 5% or sodium chloride 0.9%, and are stable for 24 hours at room temperature.

Stability in Practice
In aqueous solution, pethidine hydrolyses to pethidic acid and ethanol.[2] The rate of hydrolysis is dependent on pH, sodium chloride concentration, and temperature. In acidic conditions the reaction is first-order. Maximum stability is in the range pH 4–5.[3]

An investigation by the WHO classified pethidine as 'a less stable drug substance' in situations simulating tropical conditions.[4] Injections should be protected from light and stored at a temperature less than 40°C. The recommended maximum storage temperature is 30°C. The commercial product has a shelf-life of 36 months.

Published Information   The stability of solutions containing pethidine hydrochloride 300 mg/L in glucose 4%, glucose 5%, sodium chloride 0.18%, and sodium chloride 0.9% was studied using HPLC. Pethidine hydrochloride was found to be stable at this concentration for at least 24 hours at room temperature (approximately 25°C).[5]

Unpublished Information   Pethidine 2.5 mg/mL in sodium chloride 0.9% in PVC bags was reported to be stable for three weeks at room temperature in the light, following an investigation using GC assay. No decomposition of the drug was detected in the study period.[6]

In a similar study, the stability of pethidine 10 mg/mL in sodium chloride 0.9% in a 50 mL polypropylene syringe was assessed by HPLC and found to be stable for one month in a refrigerator (2–8°C).[7]

The chemical and physical compatibility of an analgesic combination of pethidine hydrochloride 3 mg/mL with bupivacaine 2.5 mg/mL was studied in a portable infusion device at 8°C and 37°C. The combination was found to be stable for at least 14 days under refrigerated storage and seven days at 37°C.[8]

Incompatibilities   Pethidine hydrochloride solutions have been reported to be physically or chemically incompatible with the following drug substances: aciclovir sodium; allopurinol; aminophylline; barbiturate salts; cefepime hydrochloride; cefoperazone sodium; flucloxacillin; fluopromazine; frusemide; heparin sodium; hydrocortisone sodium succinate; idarubicin; imipenem-cilastatin sodium; methicillin sodium; methylprednisolone sodium succinate; minocycline hydrochloride; morphine sulphate; nitrofurantoin sodium; nafcillin sodium; oxytetracycline hydrochloride; phenytoin sodium; potassium iodide; sulphadiazine sodium; sulphafurazole diethanolamine; tetracycline hydrochloride; thiamylal sodium; and verapamil hydrochloride.[9,10]

Compatibilities   Specialist references should be consulted for specific compatibility information.[10]

Pethidine 2.5 mg/mL with bupivacaine 1.25 mg/mL in sodium chloride 0.9% in PVC infusion containers was found to be stable for at least 24 hours at room temperature. The potency of both drugs was unchanged throughout the study with no evidence of sorption onto the PVC of the infusion bag.[11]

Comments

In common clinical practice pethidine hydrochloride is stable for 24 hours at room temperature. Little reliable information has been published on the compatibility of pethidine with other injectable drugs. Information on physical compatibility should be interpreted with care.

References

1. Bretschneider H. Osmolalities of commercially supplied drugs often used in anesthesia. Anesth Analg 1987; 66: 361-2.
2. Lund W, editor. The pharmaceutical codex: principles and practice of pharmaceutics, 12th edition. London: The Pharmaceutical Press, 1994: 993-4.
3. Patel RM, Chin T-F, Lach JL. Kinetic study of the acid hydrolysis of meperidine hydrochloride. Am J Hosp Pharm 1968; 25: 256-61.
4. WHO. WHO expert committee on specifications for pharmaceutical preparations: 31st report. WHO Tech Rep Ser 790, 1990.
5. Rudd L, Simpson P. Pethidine stability in intravenous solutions. Med J Aust 1978; 2: 34.
6. Grassby P. Personal communication, 1996.
7. Shaw RS. Personal communication, 1996.
8. Sewell GJ. Personal communication, 1996.
9. Reynolds JEF, editor. Martindale: the extra pharmacopoeia, 31st edition. London: The Pharmaceutical Press, 1996: 86-8.
10. Trissel LA. Handbook on injectable drugs, 9th edition. Bethesda, MD: American Society of Health-System Pharmacists Inc, 1996: 673-81.
11. Grassby PF, Roberts DE. Stability of epidural opiate solutions in 0.9% sodium chloride infusion bags. Int J Pharm Pract 1995; 3: 174-7.

Prepared by

Tim Sizer

Piperacillin

Approved Name

Piperacillin sodium

UK Proprietary Name

Pipril (Wyeth Laboratories)

Other Names

—

Product Details

Glass vials containing piperacillin (as the sodium salt) 1 g, 2 g, and 4 g powder for reconstitution. Also, infusion bottles containing 4 g piperacillin (as the sodium salt) powder for reconstitution with 50 mL water for injection. The injection has a pH of 5.5–7.5.[1]

Piperacillin has an osmolality of 389 mosmol/kg in glucose 5%, and 399 mosmol/kg in sodium chloride 0.9%.[2]

Preparation of Injection

For bolus administration, each gram of piperacillin should be reconstituted with 5 mL of water for injection. For infusion, piperacillin should be reconstituted as above and diluted to 50 mL with either compound sodium lactate, glucose 5%, sodium chloride 0.9%, or water for injection.

Each gram of piperacillin displaces 0.73 mL.[3]

Administration

Piperacillin may be administered by slow intravenous injection over 3–5 minutes or by infusion in at least 50 mL over 20–40 minutes.

Stability in Practice

The dry powder is stable for three years at room temperature. Exposure to light may result in a slight darkening of the powder but no loss of potency. Piperacillin is stable in solution between pH 4.5–8.5.

Published Information The manufacturer states that once reconstituted, solutions are stable for 24 hours at room temperature and 48 hours at 4°C.[4]

Another source reports that following reconstitution with glucose 5%, lignocaine 0.5–1% injection, sodium chloride 0.9%, or water for injection, piperacillin is stable in the glass vial for 24 hours at room temperature, seven days in a refrigerator (2–8°C), or one month when frozen.[5]

The stability of a piperacillin 4 g/50 mL infusion in sodium chloride 0.9% PVC minibags was reported to be 100 days at -20°C followed after thawing for four days at 5°C, and 24 hours at room temperature.[6] In the same study, storage in a refrigerator at 5°C was followed for 75 days. Results indicated that a shelf-life of 28 days at 5°C was appropriate for piperacillin sodium 80 mg/mL in sodium chloride 0.9%.[6]

The stability of piperacillin in an elastomeric infusion device was investigated by liquid chromatographic methods. Samples were stored in glucose 5% and sodium chloride 0.9% in glass vials and the latex reservoir of an elastomeric device. Piperacillin 30 mg/mL was found to be stable for at least 24 hours at 25°C, seven days at 5°C, and four weeks at -20°C.[7]

Unpublished Information In glass bottles, piperacillin 1 g/5 mL is said to retain potency for seven days at 3°C and one month if frozen at -15°C.

Piperacillin infusions, stored in plastic infusion bags at a strength of 1 g/500 mL, in either compound sodium lactate, glucose 5%, or sodium chloride 0.9% are said to be stable for two days at 25°C, 28 days at 5°C, and 71 days at -10°C.

An infusion of piperacillin 4 g/100 mL in glucose 5%, stored in minibags, has been claimed to be stable for 28 days at 5°C, with less than 5% degradation if protected from light.[8]

In plastic syringes, piperacillin 2 g/5 mL is said to be stable for two days at 25°C when reconstituted with water for injection. Chemical stability is retained for 32 days in glass and plastic syringes when frozen (temperature not stated).

Incompatibilities The compatibility of piperacillin with other drug substances depends on several factors such as, concentration, pH, diluent solution and temperature. Piperacillin has a high potential for interaction with aminoglycosides e.g. amikacin, gentamicin, netilmicin, and tobramycin. Incompatibility has also been reported with filgrastim, ondansetron, sargramostim, sodium bicarbonate, and vinorelbine tartrate.[2,5]

Piperacillin should not be mixed with blood or blood products.

Compatibilities Piperacillin is compatible with the following infusion fluids: compound sodium lactate; dextran 6% in sodium chloride 0.9%; glucose 5%; glucose 30%; mannitol 20%; and sodium chloride 0.9%.[5]

Piperacillin is also compatible with glucose 5% and sodium chloride 0.9% admixed with sodium bicarbonate.

Piperacillin is compatible and stable for 24 hours when admixed with the following drug substances in either compound sodium lactate, glucose 5%, or sodium chloride 0.9%: cefoxitin sodium; cephamandole nafate; cephazolin sodium; and flucloxacillin sodium.

A commercial product containing piperacillin 2 g, 3 g, or 4 g with tazobactam 250 mg, 375 mg, or 500 mg is available in the US.

Comments

Piperacillin has reasonable aqueous stability in the pH range 4.5–8.5. When diluted with sodium chloride 0.9%, it may be expected to retain its potency for at least seven days in a refrigerator (2–8°C) or 24 hours at room temperature.

References

1. Reynolds JEF, editor. Martindale: the extra pharmacopoeia, 31st edition. London: The Pharmaceutical Press, 1996: 262-3.
2. Trissel LA. Handbook on injectable drugs, 9th edition. Bethesda, MD: American Society of Health-System Pharmacists Inc, 1996: 891-6.
3. Mulholland P. Displacement values of powder injections. Pharm J 1993; 251: 14-5.
4. ABPI. Compendium of data sheets and summaries of product characteristics 1996-1997. London: Datapharm Publications Ltd, 1996: 1253-4.
5. McEvoy GE, editor. American hospital formulary service, drug information. Bethesda, MD: American Society of Health-System Pharmacists Inc, 1997: 891-6.
6. Brown AF, et al. Freeze-thaw stability of antibiotics used in an IV additive service. Br J Parenter Ther 1986; 7(2): 42-4.
7. Allen LV, et al. Stability of 14 drugs in the latex reservoir of an elastomeric infusion device. Am J Health-Syst Pharm 1996; 53: 2740-3.
8. Allwood M. Personal communication, 1991.

Prepared by

Krissy Cock and Tim Sizer

Teicoplanin

Approved Name

Teicoplanin

UK Proprietary Name

Targocid (Hoechst Marion Roussel Ltd)

Other Names

Teichomycin; teichomycin A_2.

Product Details

Available in packs containing a vial of a white coloured teicoplanin lyophilisate for reconstitution along with an ampoule of diluent (water for injection). Vials are available in two strengths and contain an overage of teicoplanin such that when reconstituted as directed 200 mg or 400 mg of teicoplanin is produced. The vials are preservative free. Sodium content is less than 0.5 mmol per 200 mg or 400 mg.[1,2]

Preparation of Injection

The injection should be carefully reconstituted as directed to avoid the formation of a stable foam. The entire contents of the accompanying water ampoule should slowly be added to the teicoplanin vial. The vial should then be gently rolled until the powder is completely dissolved. The vial should not be shaken. If a foam is formed the vial should be allowed to stand for 15 minutes to allow the foam to subside. The entire contents of the vial should then be slowly withdrawn into a syringe.

Administration

Teicoplanin may be administered by either intravenous or intramuscular injection. Intravenous administration may be by slow injection over five minutes or by infusion over 30 minutes. Suitable diluents include: compound sodium lactate; glucose 5%; peritoneal dialysis solution containing glucose 1.36% or 3.86%; sodium chloride 0.9%; and sodium chloride 0.18% and glucose 4%.[1-3] Continuous infusion is not usually recommended.[3]

Stability in Practice

Vials of dry teicoplanin should be stored at temperatures below 25°C.

Satisfactory potency of the reconstituted injection is retained for seven days at 4°C, and for 48 hours at 25°C.[2]

Solutions diluted with compound sodium lactate or sodium chloride 0.9% may be stored for up to seven days at 4°C; solutions left at room temperature for greater than 24 hours should be discarded.[2] The manufacturer recommends that solutions containing glucose should be stored at 4°C and used within 24 hours.[2]

Published Information Teicoplanin has become established as an alternative to vancomycin in the treatment of peritonitis associated with continuous ambulatory peritoneal dialysis (CAPD) and studies have investigated the stability of teicoplanin in dialysis solutions.[4,5] In one study,[4] the stability of teicoplanin 25 mg/L in dialysis solution containing glucose 1.36% was studied for a period of 42 days. Dialysis solutions were stored in 2L bags at 4°C, 20°C, and 37°C. Analysis was by a stability indicating bioassay with loss of more than 10% of teicoplanin activity indicative of instability. Results showed that teicoplanin stability in the dialysis solution was temperature dependent. Samples stored at 4°C were stable for the 42 day study period with a teicoplanin loss in activity of 4.6%. At 20°C teicoplanin loss was 16.8% and at 37°C, the loss was 57.8% after 42 days. Extrapolation of the data suggested a 10% loss in activity would occur after 25 days storage at 20°C and after seven days at 37°C.

A similar study of teicoplanin 25 mg/L in dialysis solution containing glucose 1.5% stored in 250 mL PVC bags showed that teicoplanin was stable following storage for 24 hours at 25°C followed by a further eight hours at 37°C. The same concentration of teicoplanin was also stable after seven days storage at 4°C followed by 16 hours at 25°C and 8 hours at 37°C. Analysis was by a stability indicating HPLC method.[5]

Unpublished Information After reconstitution, teicoplanin in the original glass vials is reported to be stable for at least 48 hours at room temperature or 21 days at 5°C. In polypropylene and high impact styrene syringes no change in potency or HPLC profile was noted over 48 hours at 4°C and 25°C. Teicoplanin in a concentration range of 1–16 mg/mL in sodium chloride 0.9% was stable for at least 21 days at 5°C in PVC infusion containers.[6]

Similarly, teicoplanin 2–10 mg/mL in glucose 5% or glucose 5% with sodium chloride 0.9%, was stable for two days at 5°C in PVC bags. In compound sodium lactate injection, teicoplanin 2 mg/mL or 4 mg/mL was stable for three days at 5°C or 30°C. When diluted with glucose 10% to a concentration of 1.2 mg/mL, teicoplanin was stable for 24 hours at room temperature (25°C).[6]

Incompatibilities Teicoplanin and aminoglycoside solutions are incompatible when mixed directly.[1] A simulated Y-site administration study has shown that teicoplanin is incompatible with ciprofloxacin.[7]

Compatibilities Teicoplanin injection is reported to be compatible with the following solutions: compound sodium lactate; glucose 5%; peritoneal dialysis solution containing glucose 1.36% or 3.86%; sodium chloride 0.9%; and sodium chloride 0.18% and glucose 4%.[1,2]

Comments

Teicoplanin when reconstituted or diluted has variable stability, depending upon the diluent and storage temperature. In clinical use, solutions should be discarded within 24 hours at room temperature.

References

1. ABPI. Compendium of data sheets and summaries of product characteristics 1996-1997. London: Datapharm Publications Ltd, 1996: 583-4.
2. Thomas J, editor. Australian prescription products guide 1997, volume 2. Hawthorn, Victoria: Australian Pharmaceutical Publishing Company Ltd, 1997: 2413-4.
3. Mehta DK, editor. British national formulary, number 33. London: British Medical Association and Royal Pharmaceutical Society of Great Britain, 1997: 611.
4. Mawhinney WM, et al. Long-term stability of teicoplanin in dialysis fluid: implications for the home-treatment of CAPD peritonitis. Int J Pharm Pract 1991; 1: 90-3.
5. Manduru M, et al. Stability of ceftazidime sodium and teicoplanin sodium in a peritoneal dialysis solution. Am J Health-Syst Pharm 1996; 53: 2731-4.
6. Marion Merrel Dow Ltd. Personal communication, 1993.
7. Jim LK. Physical and chemical compatibility of intravenous ciprofloxacin with other drugs. Ann Pharmacother 1993; 27: 704-7.

Prepared by

Tim Sizer and Paul Weller

Vancomycin

Approved Name
Vancomycin hydrochloride

UK Proprietary Name
Vancocin CP (Eli Lilly)

Other Names
—

Product Details
The proprietary preparation (Vancocin CP) consists of glass vials containing an off-white, lyophilised plug of chromatographically purified vancomycin. It is available as 250000i.u., 500000i.u., or 1000000i.u., equivalent to 250mg, 500mg, and 1g respectively. When reconstituted in water, it forms a clear solution with a pH between 2.8–4.5. If more accurate reconstitution is required, the displacement value is 0.3mL/500mg.[1]

Another preparation (Faulding Pharmaceuticals) is available as freeze-dried powder in glass vials containing either vancomycin 500mg or 1g.

Preparation of Injection
Vancomycin 250mg should be reconstituted with 5mL of water for injection, vancomycin 500mg with 10mL of water for injection, and vancomycin 1g with 20mL of water for injection. The resulting 50mg/mL solution should be further diluted prior to intravenous infusion.[2]

Administration
The preferred method of administration is intermittent intravenous infusion. The required dose should be added to 100–200mL of glucose 5% or sodium chloride 0.9% infusion solution and infused at no more than 10mg/min.

Stability in Practice
Vancomycin vials should be stored at or below 25°C and protected from light. The manufacturers state that when aseptically prepared, the product may be stored for up to 24 hours at 2–8°C. However, as the product is not microbially preserved, if aseptic preparation cannot be assured, the product should be prepared immediately before use.[2]

Published Information Vancomycin is a tricyclic glycopeptide antibiotic used to treat gram-positive bacterial infections. It has been found to be fairly stable in commonly used solutions and is most stable at pH 3–5.[3]

In both two and three piece syringes, at a concentration of 10mg/mL in glucose 5%, sodium chloride 0.9%, or water for injection, vancomycin has been shown to be stable for at least 84 days at 4°C. At 25°C, stability was greater than 28 days, although more varied between syringe types and diluents, being most stable in sodium chloride 0.9% in a three piece polypropylene syringe.[4]

Admixtures in glucose 5% and sodium chloride 0.9% in PVC bags have been shown to be stable for 14 days and 21 days respectively at 23°C, and for 24 days and 30 days respectively at 4°C. The concentrations studied were 4 and 5mg/mL.[5] It has been reported that vancomycin 5mg/mL solutions were stable for at least 63 days at -10°C and 5°C in glass vials, and 17 days at 24°C in glass vials or PVC bags.[6]

In another study, stability of vancomycin 5mg/mL and 8mg/mL solutions were studied in PVC infusion bags. In both glucose 5% and sodium chloride 0.9%, no significant degradation was observed either after 48 hours at 22°C, without protection from light, or after seven days at 4°C with protection from light. There was also no leaching of di-ethyl hexyl phthalate (DEHP) from the PVC detected.[7]

A vancomycin 5mg/mL solution in an elastomeric infusion device has been shown to be stable for at least 24 hours at 25°C, 14 days at 4°C, and nine weeks at -20°C. This was found using both glucose 5% and sodium chloride 0.9% as diluents.[8]

It has been shown that vancomycin can be safely stored in portable infusion pump reservoirs, prior to administration, for 24 hours at 5°C or 30°C.[9] A study using a biological assay method showed that a vancomycin 500mg/100mL solution in glucose 5% maintained adequate antibiotic activity for at least 28 days when stored at either 5°C or 25°C. However, in sodium chloride 0.9%, activity was maintained for at least 28 days when stored at 5°C, but for less than 28 days at 25°C.[10]

Unpublished information A vancomycin 50mg/ mL solution in sodium chloride 0.9% contained in a three piece 2 mL syringe was found to be stable for at least 56 days when refrigerated and for at least 28 days at room temperature.[11] Similarly, a vancomycin 5 mg/mL solution in sodium chloride 0.9% in a three piece syringe was found to be stable for at least 26 days at both 4°C and 20°C.[12]

Incompatibilities As vancomycin is stable only in acid pH, there is a wide range of alkaline drugs with which it is incompatible. Vancomycin has been reported to be chemically or physically incompatible with the following drug substances: aminophylline; ceftazidime;[13] chloramphenicol; dexamethasone sodium phosphate; heparin sodium; idarubicin;[14] methicillin sodium; phenobarbitone sodium and other barbiturates; sodium bicarbonate;[2] and warfarin sodium.

Although a study found cefotaxime to be compatible with vancomycin,[7] cefotaxime has been shown to be incompatible with vancomycin sulphate.[15]

Compatibilities Specialist references should be consulted for specific compatibility information, including compatibility with peritoneal dialysis fluids.[14] Vancomycin hydrochloride has been shown to be physically and chemically compatible with aztreonam, in glucose 5% or sodium chloride 0.9%, at concentrations of 1 mg/mL and 4 mg/mL respectively, for seven days at 32°C and significantly longer at lower temperatures, but not at higher concentrations.[16]

Comments

Vancomycin hydrochloride has been shown to be stable for a number of days in both glucose 5% and sodium chloride 0.9% in a range of standard injectable containers. However, because it is most stable in quite acid conditions, mixing with other drugs should be approached with great care.

References

1. Mulholland P. Displacement values of powder injections. Pharm J 1993; 251: 14-5.
2. ABPI. Compendium of data sheets and summaries of product characteristics 1996-1997. London: Datapharm Publications Ltd, 1996: 349-50, 539-40.
3. Mann JM, Coleman DL, Boylan JC. Stability of parenteral solutions of sodium cephalothin, cephaloridine, potassium penicillin G (buffered) and vancomycin hydrochloride. Am J Hosp Pharm 1971; 28: 760-3.
4. Wood MJ, Lund R, Beavan M. Stability of vancomycin in plastic syringes measured by high-performance liquid chromatography. J Clin Pharm Ther 1995; 20: 319-25.
5. Walker SE, Birkhans B. Stability of intravenous vancomycin. Can J Hosp Pharm 1988; 41: 233-42.
6. Das Gupta V, Stewart KR, Nohria S. Stability of vancomycin hydrochloride in 5% dextrose and 0.9% sodium chloride injections. Am J Hosp Pharm 1986; 43: 1729-31.
7. Khalfi F, et al. Compatibility and stability of vancomycin hydrochloride with PVC infusion material in various conditions using stability-indicating high-performance liquid chromatographic assay. Int J Pharmaceutics 1996; 139: 243-7.
8. Allen LV, et al. Stability of 14 drugs in the latex reservoir of an elastomeric infusion device. Am J Health-Syst Pharm 1996; 53: 2740-3.
9. Stiles ML, Allen LV, Prince SJ. Stability of various antibiotics kept in an insulated pouch during administration via portable infusion pump. Am J Health-Syst Pharm 1995; 52: 70-4.
10. Mann JM, Coleman DL, Boylan JC. Stability of parenteral solutions of sodium cephalothin, cephaloridine, potassium penicillin G (buffered) and vancomycin hydrochloride. Am J Hosp Pharm 1971; 28: 760-3.
11. Walker J. Personal communication, 1996.
12. Haines-Nutt F. Personal Communication, 1998.
13. Cairns CJ, Robertson J. Incompatibility of ceftazidime and vancomycin. Pharm J 1987; 238: 577.
14. Trissel LA. Handbook on injectable drugs, 9th edition. Bethesda, MD: American Society of Health-System Pharmacists Inc, 1996: 1072-8.
15. Szof C, Walker PC. Incompatibility of cefotaxime sodium and vancomycin sulfate during Y-site administration. Am J Hosp Pharm 1993; 50: 2054, 2057.
16. Trissel LA, Xu QA, Martinez JF. Compatibility and stability of aztreonam and vancomycin hydrochloride. Am J Health-Syst Pharm 1995; 52: 2560-4.

Prepared by

Richard Needle

Zidovudine

Approved Name
Zidovudine

UK Proprietary Name
Retrovir (Glaxo Wellcome)

Other Names
Azidothymidine; AZT.

Product Details
Vials containing zidovudine 200 mg in 20 mL of sterile aqueous solution; pH is approximately 5.5.[1]

Preparation of Injection
The injection must be diluted prior to administration. The required dose should be mixed with glucose 5% to give a final zidovudine concentration of either 2 mg/mL or 4 mg/mL.[1]

Administration
Administration should be by slow intravenous infusion over a one-hour period. [1]

Stability in Practice
The manufacturer indicates that the injection is stable for up to 48 hours at both 5°C and 25°C when diluted as specified above.[1]

Published Information The chemical stability of zidovudine was investigated in glucose 5% and sodium chloride 0.9% injections (250 mL PVC bags) at a concentration of 4 mg/mL. Analysis was by stability indicating HPLC assay. Storage was at 4°C and 25°C for up to eight days. Results indicated no detectable loss of zidovudine at 4°C or 25°C after eight days storage in PVC bags. No substantial change in pH was observed in any solution. There was no visible evidence of any precipitation or colour change during the study at either 4°C or 25°C.[2]

Compatibilities Studies have been published in which the physical stability of zidovudine 4 mg/mL was assessed in combination with a range of drugs in a simulated Y-site injection.[3,4] In all cases, physical compatibility was apparent at room temperature for four hours; chemical compatibility was not assessed.

Comments
The above studies indicate that zidovudine 4 mg/mL in glucose 5% and sodium chloride 0.9% infusions stored in PVC bags are stable, and compatible, for up to eight days at 4°C or 25°C. The chemical stability of zidovudine in combination with other drugs needs to be assessed in order to provide robust guidance on drug admixtures.

References
1. ABPI. Compendium of data sheets and summaries of product characteristics 1996-97. London: Datapharm Publications Ltd, 1996: 1206-8.
2. Lam NP, et al. Stability of zidovudine in 5% dextrose injection and 0.9% sodium chloride injection. Am J Hosp Pharm 1991; 48: 280-2.
3. Trissel LA. Handbook on injectable Drugs, 9th edition. Bethesda, MD: American Society of Health-System Pharmacists Inc, 1996: 1107-10.
4. Bashaw ED, et al. Visual compatibility of zidovudine with other injectable drugs during simulated Y-site administration. Am J Hosp Pharm 1988; 45: 2532-3.

Prepared by
Steve Brown

Index